WHAT *to* EAT
if YOU HAVE
DIABETES

WHAT *to* EAT *if* YOU HAVE DIABETES

A Guide to Adding Nutritional Therapy to Your Treatment Plan

MAUREEN KEANE, M.S., AND
DANIELLA CHACE, M.S.

CB
CONTEMPORARY BOOKS

Library of Congress Cataloging-in-Publication Data

Keane, Maureen.
    What to eat if you have diabetes : a guide to adding
nutritional therapy to your treatment plan / Maureen
Keane and Daniella Chace.
        p.   cm.
    Includes bibliographical references.
    ISBN 0-8092-2966-8
    1. Diabetes—Diet therapy.   I. Chace, Daniella.
II. Title.
RC662.K43   1998
616.4'620654—dc21   98-3869
                                             CIP

Disclaimer
The following approaches have been shown to help people who
have been diagnosed with diabetes. This book is not meant to
replace medical care but to be used as an adjunct to medical
treatment. Check with your doctor before changing your diet or
dosage of pills or insulin. You and your medical team will need to
work out a program especially for you.

Cover design by Kim Bartko
Cover image: Charlotte Segal, *Valley of the Gods*. Diptych, oil on paper.
Copyright © Charlotte Segal. Used with permission of the artist.
Photo: James Prinz Photography, Chicago
Interior design by Mary Lockwood
Interior illustrations by David Stevenson

Published by Contemporary Books
A division of NTC/Contemporary Publishing Group, Inc.
4255 West Touhy Avenue, Lincolnwood (Chicago), Illinois 60712-1975 U.S.A.
Copyright © 1999 by Daniella Chace and Maureen B. Keane
All rights reserved. No part of this book may be reproduced, stored in a retrieval
system, or transmitted in any form or by any means, electronic, mechanical,
photocopying, recording, or otherwise, without the prior written permission of
NTC/Contemporary Publishing Group, Inc.
Printed in the United States of America
International Standard Book Number: 0-8092-2966-8
99 00 01 02 03 04 QP 19 18 17 16 15 14 13 12 11 10 9 8 7 6 5 4 3 2

This book is dedicated to
Daniella's sister Darcie
in gratitude for helping us
better understand the realities
of living with diabetes and
eating well.

Contents

Foreword

$\mathcal{D}$iabetes is a disorder of sugar metabolism that affects millions of Americans. Although the cause of diabetes is not completely understood, it usually involves either a deficiency of insulin (a blood sugar–lowering hormone from the pancreas) or a failure of insulin to do its job properly in the body (insulin resistance). Individuals with diabetes are at high risk of developing serious complications, including heart and blood vessel disease; damage to the eyes, kidneys, and nervous system; and reduced ability to fight infections.

There is considerable scientific evidence that dietary modification can reduce and sometimes completely normalize elevated blood sugar levels in diabetics. That is important, because maintaining blood sugar close to or within the normal range may reduce the risk of complications developing. In addition, specific nutritional supplements have been shown to improve blood sugar control and may also help prevent some of the organ damage that results from diabetes.

In this book, Daniella Chace and Maureen B. Keane present an easy-to-understand overview of this common medical condition. They also describe the dietary changes and individual nutrients that may be beneficial for diabetics. Of particular importance is their discussion about foods that are high in fiber and complex carbohydrates. Diabetics who incorporate these types of foods into their diet often experience a reduction in blood sugar and may be able to reduce the dosage of their diabetes medication.

The information in this book is important for most people who struggle with diabetes. It should be noted, however, that diabetes should be treated only under medical supervision.

While dietary changes and nutritional supplements may be helpful in the long run, they might also influence medication requirements. People who fail to lower their medication dosages appropriately could develop a potentially dangerous fall in blood sugar levels. In addition, some individuals with long-standing diabetes have already developed kidney damage; in such cases, a high-fiber diet might actually result in a dangerous buildup of potassium in the body. On the other hand, if a doctor monitors a diabetic's nutritional program, the potential benefits are enormous.

Alan R. Gaby, M.D.
Past President, American Holistic Medical Association
Professor of Nutrition, Bastyr University

Preface

*W*hen she was twenty-one, my sister was diagnosed with diabetes mellitus. Our family doctor wanted her to start taking insulin injections immediately. Darcie's blood sugar levels were sporadic. Our mother, Linda, who is constantly at work to make our lives just a little easier, would not accept this without a fight. She knew the dangers and complications of taking insulin and began reading all the studies she could find regarding treating diabetes naturally. She set to work interviewing doctors in hopes of finding alternatives.

She spoke with naturopathic doctors, nutritionists, and dietitians. She read case studies of patients whose diabetes were halted or reversed with a high-carbohydrate, leguminous diet. These led her to the research of Dr. James Anderson, who had developed a diabetic diet based on plant protein from beans. Many of his patients were able to stabilize their blood sugar with this one simple change in their diets—eating more beans. These patients could reduce the amount of insulin they needed to take.

Beans were not a part of our meals, so Mom found legume recipes and began testing and tailoring them to meet my sister's tastes. Darcie, you see, lives for apple pie and deep-fried chicken. She craved the fast food that was promoted on TV and that everyone else was eating. I remember her scrunching up her nose in rejection at bean soups and lentil burgers and crying when she was told she could not have a piece of her own birthday cake.

Somehow, through unrelenting persistence and a whole lot of love, our mother made beans acceptable. Darcie finally started eating some beans each day. We were delighted to find that her blood sugar levels remained within normal range. After several months Darcie thought maybe she was out of the woods and began to slip on her diet. She started eating fast food and cut back on her consumption of beans. Soon her blood sugar began to crawl back up. This culminated in a visit to the hospital, where her doctor started insulin shots and told her she would have to take them the rest of her life.

Darcie needed insulin at that point, and I am thankful that we have this miracle of medicine. But I was left to ponder whether she would have ever had to start taking insulin if she had continued to eat beans each day. My mind was opened to the possibilities of nutrition as an adjunct to treatment for diabetes.

Over the next few years, I watched her blood sugar stabilize when she ate beans and included supplements such as magnesium, chromium, and vitamin C. We learned so much in those experimental years, with Darcie as our begrudging subject to lead us on our path of discovery. We saw how the wrong foods made her ill. When her blood sugar level went up she became more dehydrated, which raised her readings even higher. We also noticed her sugar level drop dramatically when she simply rehydrated with water. We saw her blood sugar levels jump past 300 milligrams per deciliter on several occasions after she drank diet sodas alone. And we learned that a can of olives does not count as a vegetable serving. That can of "vegetables" sent her to the hospital with a sugar level of 700.

But we also learned that beans are stabilizing and that taking a chromium supplement assuaged Darcie's headaches immediately. We learned that you can take a whole lot less insulin if you are exercising regularly and that stress alone can throw your blood sugar out of balance.

If you or a loved one has diabetes, then you are very lucky if you have an angel like our mother to watch out for you. But if you don't you can be your own angel. Diabetes is your cue to get healthy and do whatever it takes to avoid developing complications. The really good news is that although diabetes is a complicated physiological disease, it can be controlled so that you will feel well again. The primary therapy for blood sugar disorders is diet. Whether you are taking insulin or just experiencing hypoglycemia, you will benefit from eating fresh whole plant foods, getting some exercise, and taking the appropriate supplements.

Your meal plan can be made of delicious foods. For example, whole-grain cereal, raspberry vanilla smoothies, bean dip, marinated tuna, lentil and arame stew, roasted eggplant and mozzarella sandwiches, and chocolate mousse are included in this meal plan therapy (recipes in *The What to Eat if You Have Diabetes Cookbook*). You will be eating the same types of foods that supermodels who want to stay slim and athletes who want to gain muscle eat. The nutrient-dense, high-fiber choices that make up the core of the foods for this meal plan will also reduce your chances of developing heart disease, circulatory complications, eye problems, hypertension, cancer, and arthritis.

The individualized health plan will guide you through the process of being your own blood sugar detective. Watch for clues that help you understand why your blood sugar fluctuates, and soon you will know how to make the little changes that will help you control your blood sugar and feel healthier.

I wish I could be there to be the angel for each of you on your journey. Enjoy your "therapy"—and watch out for those olives.

Daniella Chace

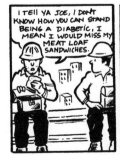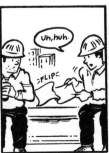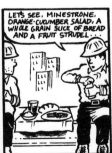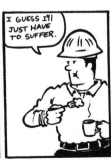

Acknowledgments

Daniella wishes to thank the following friends, family, and colleagues for their input, research, computer help, advice, and support: Linda Kay Landkamer, LaMar Harrington, Merrilee Gomez, Manuel Gomez, Nuria Gomez, Tom Gomez, Marcus Wojcik, Sally Rockwell, Suzanne Myer, David Butler, Julie Mermelstein, Michelle LaRock, Tara Hubbard, Jennifer James, Gary Boyer, Dave Stevenson, and Heidi Bresnahan.

Introduction

*D*iabetes mellitus (DM) directly affects about sixteen million Americans and eighty million indirectly, and this number is growing at an alarming rate. As a society we pay a high price for this largely avoidable epidemic in medical costs, lost wages, energy, and time. In this book we will present the most current theories, research, and nutritional treatment of diabetes and hypoglycemia. We will introduce you to the tools for developing an individually tailored program that includes your own health-care team, a diet of nutritionally rich and satisfying meals, the proper vitamin and mineral supplementation, and an exercise program that is right for you.

The first part of the book takes an in-depth look at the amazing machines we live in—our bodies. Some of you may choose to skip over this part of the book and head straight to Part II where you learn to develop a nutritional therapy regimen just for you. But those of you who are curious and inquisitive about your own bodies may want to take the time to read Part I. In Part I we will take you on a tour of your body, introducing you to the microscopic world inside you, to your cells, tissues, organs, organ systems all the way through to the transportation of nutrients through your bloodstream. Understanding your own anatomy and physiology will help you see the profound difference food choices make in fueling your body so that it will run well for you.

Choosing the best foods for blood sugar regulation can help those who have a predisposition to diabetes and/or hypoglycemia avoid developing the disease. Those with type 2 diabetes may even be able to reverse their metabolic disorder. Those with type 1 diabetes who are already taking insulin will find they have better control and fewer complications with this individualized program. Regulating blood sugar with diet greatly reduces the need for corrective medical procedures, such as retinal surgery, amputations, neutral therapy, organ transplants, and dialysis. Proper supplementation may help prevent such complications of diabetes as neuropathy, retinopathy, nephropathy, micro- and macroangiopathy, and cataracts. (*Alternative Medicine Review* 1997)

Part III is organized into short reference chapters, allowing you to tailor the information to your needs by reading the material that directly applies to you. For example, you may want to set up your exercise program immediately so you would read Chapter 14 today. If you smoke or drink coffee or alcohol, you will want to read Chapter 20, which covers these issues specifically. Before going to the grocery store you may want to read Chapter 16, which explains food labels, or Chapter 22, which discusses phytochemicals and blood sugar regulation, and make a note to pick up more garlic or try licorice, bitter melon, fenugreek, and holy basil. Also there are topics that may not apply to you now but may in the future, such as food allergies and candida, which often develop after a period of uncontrolled blood sugar. Use this part of the book as a reference guide to fill in the parts of your individualized program as you see fit.

With this solid education in the care and maintenance of DM you have the knowledge to reduce the ravages of disordered blood sugar and begin the journey to wellness.

WHAT *to* EAT
if YOU HAVE
DIABETES

Part I

The Body, Diabetes, and Nutrition

I

What Is Diabetes?

*T*ype 1 **diabetes** usually occurs in children, adolescents, and young adults, although it can strike at any age. This type affects approximately one out of six hundred school-age children in the United States. People with type 1 diabetes cannot produce insulin or have reduced secretion of insulin from the beta cells of the pancreas. These individuals must take insulin injections. It is estimated that insulin-dependent diabetes makes up about 3 to 5 percent of all cases. (Mertz 1993) The symptoms include excessive thirst, frequent urination, irritability, nausea, hunger, weight loss in spite of large amounts of food eaten, and ketone production. When body fat is burned as an alternative fuel, by-products called ketone bodies are created as a source of energy. Ketones cause accumulation of acids in the blood and a state of ketoacidosis, which disturbs the system's ability to maintain blood glucose balance.

Type 2 diabetes generally occurs in adults, often those who are overweight and have developed insulin resistance. This type makes up 90 percent of the cases of diabetes. In type 2 diabetes, the pancreas produces some insulin, but either it is not enough or it is simply used ineffectively. Eighty percent of people with type 2 are overweight at the time of diagnosis. Weight loss, exercise, and proper meal planning can usually control and reverse this type of diabetes. As in type 1, nutrition management is the key element to the therapy. A meal plan featuring whole plant foods is the most protective step in preventing type 2 diabetes from developing into type 1 diabetes. (Mooradian and Morley 1987, Mann 1985)

3

Less Common Types of Diabetes

A new classification of diabetes is *type 1 (noninsulin-requiring)*. People with this type are not obese and do not require insulin yet, but they do have islet-cell antibodies (ICAS). This group is at great risk of developing type 1 insulin-dependent diabetes. The destruction of the islet cells occurs gradually over time, delaying the development of the need for insulin.

People who are more than 20 percent over their ideal body weight (IBW) and have deficiencies in insulin binding sites on target cells stemming from their obesity, have *type 2A obese diabetes*. The number of insulin receptors and/or the receptors' affinity for insulin is affected in these individuals. Generally, when insulin levels in the blood are high, the plasma membrane of the cells reacts to protect the body from dangerously high levels of insulin binding. This reduces glucose absorption and thus the number of insulin receptors. The term replaces the terms *borderline*, *chemical*, and *latent diabetes*. This condition is treated with an appropriate meal plan for weight loss, if necessary, to prevent it from developing into diabetes. Type 2A obese patients benefit from the whole-foods meal plan.

2

···

Anatomy and Physiology

*P*erhaps you thought you were just feeling the symptoms of a stressful life when you found yourself needing to sleep a little longer and urinate a little more frequently. Maybe you knew to watch for the telltale signs of diabetes because you've been caring for a loved one with the disease already. Whatever your life circumstances are, your diagnosis of diabetes requires certain changes in your habits and lifestyle to regain as much control of your health as possible. Knowledge is power and, in dealing with disease, it is important to learn how to work with your body's intelligence to achieve a healthful and fulfilling life.

To reach that goal, this chapter provides some basic information about your body and how it works. Intended as a reference tool, it emphasizes the areas and systems of the body most related to diabetes.

The Microscopic World Inside You

The starting point is the tiny world of the cells. Our bodies are well-organized factories with no job or labor shortage when they are functioning optimally. You are the CEO of your factory, in charge of centralizing data and making decisions to maintain smooth operations. You must oversee the communications networks, facilitate the transportation of goods, make sure that your workers are nourished with food and water, and remove waste to keep the factory running smoothly. You must also have a cell team trained and ready to defend your company from possible hostile takeovers. Your abilities to both oversee and delegate are essential to the health and function of your factory at all times.

As the CEO, you know that each and every cell worker has a unique and vital job to perform in your company. There is no expendable worker and there is no inferior job in your factory. You know that is true whether you are dealing with the department of engineering, transportation, or sanitation. The ability of the whole team to function well together is what counts.

Organization at the Cellular Level

To understand the body activities essential to life and the origin of disease, we must first look at the cellular level of organization. Through the years we have continued to be surprised and awed by the complexities of this most basic, living, structural, and functional unit of the body: the cell. Each cell functions as an individual, self-contained worker, while manufacturing and trading goods with neighboring cells.

The cell is contained by an incredibly thin structure that serves to separate the parts inside (intracellular) from the parts outside (extracellular). This structure is called the **plasma membrane**. On the outside of the plasma membrane are many attached protein molecules that aid in communication with other body cells and foreign cells or substances. Some molecules act like little mailboxes, receiving packages of hormones, nutrients, enzymes, neurotransmitters, and antibodies. They are called **receptor sites**. The plasma membrane also performs the functions of a guard, determining what substances to allow in and what to keep out. This selective permeability can be active or passive, requiring energy or not, depending on several factors. Small molecules and water can move into the cell without effort. So can fat- (lipid-) soluble substances such as oxygen, carbon dioxide, and steroid hormones. Various sugars are also easily taken into the cells, but they require the assistance of an escort called a *carrier molecule*. In the cells of the digestive tract, however, simple sugars require energy from the cell to get in, like a special pass.

Inside the plasma membrane is a fluid in which other cellular components are found. This fluid (75 to 90 percent water), called *cytoplasm*, is a thick and elastic scaffolding that provides shape, support, protection, and communication to all structures and functions within the cell.

The structures embedded and suspended in the cytoplasm are called **organelles**. These are much like miniature organs of the body, each one performing a unique and specialized function related to growth, repair, maintenance, and control. Different cells contain different amounts and types of organelles according to each cell's function.

The largest structure in the cell is also its "brain" (or headquarters) and is called the **nucleus**. The only cells that don't contain a nucleus are mature red blood cells. Some cells even have more than one. The nucleus separates itself from the cytoplasm by a double plasma membrane called the *nuclear membrane*. The instruction manual for every cell is written out in code on structures called *chromatids*. These codes are formed from the genetic material known as DNA **(deoxyribonucleic acid)**. They determine everything from the color of your eyes to the shape of your little toe. If your DNA tells your pancreas to stop producing insulin, you will have diabetes.

Inside the cytoplasm is a system of membrane-lined channels connecting the outer plasma membrane to the inner nuclear membrane. This system is called the ER **(endoplasmic reticulum)**. Through the channels of the ER, various substances are transported, stored, and exchanged around the cell. Tiny round granules called *ribosomes* line some of the canals, making them rough and creating places for protein manufacturing.

Near the nucleus sits a structure called the *Golgi complex*. It's a complex because it's really a series of flat membranous sacs stacked on each other. The proteins that were made in the ER and moved into the Golgi complex as carbohydrates are added to form *glycoproteins*. As these glycoproteins move through the complex, they are changed according to what their function will be and where they are to go. Some become *secretory granules*, which move to the surface of the cell, break open, and release any of several substances, perhaps sweat or digestive juices. Another little sack that pinches off from the Golgi complex is called a *lysosome*. It plays a part in defending the cell from invasions by foreign substances, such as bacteria, by surrounding and consuming them.

The powerhouse of the cell is not located in a single power plant. It is found in rounded, rod-shaped organelles called **mitochondria**. These double plasma membranous structures have a smooth outer membrane and a highly folded inner one. Because of these intricate folding patterns, there is a great deal of surface area for chemical reactions to take place. This is the site of cellular respiration; here more than five hundred enzymes are involved in energy-releasing activities. You can imagine that the more active cells such as liver, muscle, and kidney have large numbers of mitochondria to keep up with the energy needed to function. Mitochondria are able to self-replicate (reproduce themselves) in response to an increase in cellular need because they contain their own DNA to do so. Because the mitochondria are relatively self-contained, scientists speculate that they are actually the descendants of bacteria that were engulfed billions of years ago by larger cells but remained undigested.

Cell Division

Just as you have a variety of cells that are assigned different duties in the function of the body, these cells have different life spans to correspond with those tasks. In addition, cells wear out, become damaged or diseased, and need to be replaced. Young people need cells to grow; older people generally need more replacements.

In order to reproduce, a cell divides in both the nucleus and the cytoplasm. There are two distinct ways in which nuclear division occurs: *meiosis* (reproductive cell division) and *mitosis* (somatic cell division). In meiosis, new sperm and egg cells are produced in preparation for a new organism. In mitosis, a parent cell divides to produce a pair of identical twin daughter cells. This ensures that all of the daughter cells contain the same encoded genetic material as the parent cell. These cells divide when their neighboring cell workers pass on the message to do so. Cells that line the **gastrointestinal (GI) tract** are continually being replaced, while cells of the nervous tissues (neurons) are programmed for life.

The large, round nucleus is the center of cell division because it is where all the programmed information resides. This information (genetic material) is found in the **chromosome**, a coiled molecule that is partially covered with DNA. The actual encoded messages are in units called **genes**.

The DNA molecule is called a double helix because its structure resembles a spiraling ladder. The ladder is constructed of sugars (*deoxyriboses*) and *phosphates* as the supports and bases for the rungs. The bases are paired and their connection is weak in the center. As the cell divides, the rungs of the ladder come apart after each chromosome has made a duplicate of itself. Then the cell cytoplasm and cell membrane both divide into two, with equal amounts of chromosomes in each half.

In summary, cells have internal structures that resemble a miniature version of your body. These cell structures, called organelles, have specific functions within the cell. They must also relate to the other cells as directed by the nucleus. When a body cell divides, the genetic information contained in the nucleus duplicates itself and then the whole cell divides in two. Your cells require energy to function, stay healthy, and reproduce.

Tissues

Cells group together to form a community of cells around a common function. These physically similar cells with the same encoded message to perform a specialized activity are called

tissues. Epithelial, connective, muscular, and nervous tissue are the four principal types of tissues found in the human body. Each tissue type has different types of cells, arranged in different patterns relating to their function and their location. Cells on the outside of your body need to be stronger and more durable, so they are generally stacked in several layers. Other specialized cells have a loosely woven pattern to allow for stretching and movement. Still others are designed to be extremely sensitive to stimuli.

Epithelial Tissue

Epithelial tissue is the cells that make up the shape that you see as you. They make contact with everything outside your body. They also line your body cavities, protecting you against adversaries and the natural elements, keeping your skin from drying out, cushioning the underlying tissues, and secreting substances that help the body to function. These tissues cover and line your blood vessels, heart, respiratory system, and digestive tract.

The cells of the epithelial tissue are found in a variety of shapes according to their function. The tissues are made up of layers of tightly packed, single cells that resemble thin, delicate sheets. The sheets are single or multilayered and connect at the plasma membranes of the cells. The sheets are then connected to the underlying connective tissue by a thin layer called the *basement membrane*. Epithelial tissue is subjected to enough injury, wear, and tear that it needs to be able to reproduce itself rapidly. This is the tissue that designer Band-Aids were made for!

Connective Tissue

Connective tissue is the type you have the most of in your body. Connective tissue is highly versatile, like a worker with many trades. Its functions are binding, supporting, connecting, separating, transporting, and protecting. The cells of connective tissue (except for cartilage) are not densely packed like those of epithelial tissues. Connective tissue cells are scattered, leaving plenty of room for intercellular substances. The intercellular substance determines the quality of the tissue and can be anything from fluid (like blood) to highly fibrous tissue (like bone). The cells of connective tissue also protect you by forming antibodies and ingesting bacteria or cell debris. By storing fat, connective tissue holds energy in reserve.

Muscle Tissue

Muscular tissues are highly specialized for contraction. This means movement as well as the production of heat and the maintenance of posture. There are three types of muscle tissue, classified by their functions and structures. *Skeletal muscle tissue* attaches to bone. This tissue is called voluntary because you can tell it to contract or relax. *Cardiac muscle tissue*, on the other hand, is usually involuntary. The fibers of muscle tissue are uniquely bound together to add strength and promote quick, strong contraction. This tissue makes up the bulk of the wall of your heart. *Smooth (visceral) muscle tissue* is also involuntary. It forms the walls of structures such as the blood vessels, stomach, and intestines.

Nervous Tissue

The cells of the nervous tissues are highly specialized for sensitivity. The structural and functional cells are called *neurons*. They conduct nerve impulses (electrical communications) to neighboring cells, tissues, organs, and organ systems. *Neuroglia cells* connect and support the neurons.

To recap, cells group together around a common function, much as a labor union organizes around a common cause. They group into a specific shape and size according to the task they are assigned to perform. The job of the epithelial tissue is to cover, line, secrete, and absorb. Connective tissue supports, connects, separates, transports, and protects from hostile takeovers. The task of movement is left to the muscle tissue, and communication is the specialty of the nervous tissue.

Organs and Organ Systems

When tissues group together to perform a specific function, they are referred to as an **organ**. Organs working together to accomplish specialized tasks in the body are called an **organ system**. Just as the cells of an organ rely on one another to accomplish their task, so do the organs within a system depend on the optimal functioning of one another. The organs most directly involved with diabetes and hypoglycemia are the liver and the pancreas. The digestive system and endocrine system are the most acutely affected systems of the body.

These distinctions are helpful in describing how the body works, but it is not really partitioned into segments and components. The entire body functions as a system on the highest level of organization. So, while we talk about the levels of organization separately, it is important to bear in mind that they are always working together in an interconnected relationship. In order for a leg bone to move, it must have a muscle attached. But first it must have a signal from the communication system, and so on. Each system relies on the others to maintain *homeostasis* (balance) in structure and function.

The Integumentary System

Integumentary system is a long way to say skin. This is actually the largest organ of the body by surface area because it also includes hair, nails, glands, and some specialized receptor cells. This system performs several functions that are essential to your survival. The cells that work here are the security guards of your factory. They keep the worker cells in and the bacteria out. They protect you from ultraviolet radiation. Without skin, the underlying tissues would **dehydrate** and be scraped by everything that touched you.

Besides the physical barrier protection of the skin, there are cells that produce antibodies that work with the immune system to fight disease. These cells assist the helper T cells or interact with suppressor T cells to protect your body.

In addition to protection, the integumentary system is responsible for temperature regulation of your factory. When the temperature is too high, the sweat glands are turned on to bring it back to the comfort zone. This not only helps to regulate your body temperature but also rids the body of water, salts, and some organic compounds. Blood flow can also be altered to make temperature adjustments. To sense external temperature, the skin contains nerve endings that communicate to the brain information about touch, pressure, and pain.

Small amounts of sunshine aid in the synthesis of vitamin D. This process starts in the skin and is very important for the absorption of calcium and phosphorus from foods, the stuff from which strong bones are made and nerve messages are sent. The liver and kidneys play an essential role in the synthesis of vitamin D. It is important to remember that these organs are highly stressed in diabetes and that stress can impair their function in a variety of ways.

Sometimes the stress of diabetes shows up as a problem with your skin. Circulation can become sluggish, as can the response of white cells that are supposed to attack invasive bacteria and germs. This can lead to a higher incidence of boils, styes, and inflammations, particularly in the feet and legs. It can also cause dry or itchy skin. Women are often subject to more frequent vaginal yeast and fungal infections. In fact, all warm, moist places in the bodies of both men and women are possible sites of fungal infections. Sometimes spots appear on the skin or ulcers from a minor problem left unattended.

The most important solution is gaining control of your blood sugar. Once that is achieved, the symptoms appearing on your skin will likely subside.

The Skeletal System

Without the skeletal system, you would probably resemble an advanced jellyfish. The skeleton holds you up and protects all that's inside your factory body. This system includes both the bones, which provide a framework, and the cartilage, which cushions the movement of one bone against another. Your skull, arm and leg bones, rib cage, joints, tendons, and ligaments are all part of this system.

In addition to support, protection, and movement, bones are a storage facility. Minerals, such as calcium and phosphorus, are stored here for use when needed by the body. Some bones produce and store red blood cells; some store white cells and platelets.

To maintain healthy bones, you *must* get enough exercise. The stress of moderate exercise causes bone to grow and slows down bone destruction by specialized body cells. Diabetes can be highly fatiguing and cause a lack of desire to exercise. *Proper regulation of blood sugar and meal plan* can help you overcome the obstacle of fatigue and low energy.

The Muscular System

In order to move your bones, make your heart beat, and push your food through your intestines, you rely on your muscle tissues. The muscular system provides motion and heat and maintains your posture.

Skeletal muscle tissue is mainly attached to bones. It is voluntary because you can tell it when to contract and relax to move a body part. Cardiac muscle tissue is similar in some ways to skeletal muscle tissue, but it is largely involuntarily controlled. It forms the walls of the heart. Smooth muscle tissue is also involuntary and automatic. Smooth muscles form the walls of the stomach, blood vessels, and intestines. There is also smooth muscle attached to hair follicles.

Nerve impulses and hormones move muscle tissue. Any muscle contraction requires a certain amount of energy. A skeletal muscle fiber can exert energy for only about five to six seconds, so more must be generated from another source. Skeletal muscle fibers contain a high-energy molecule that can break down and release quick energy for short bursts (about fifteen seconds).

The next source of energy is **glucose**, taken from the breakdown of **glycogen** and also pulled from the blood. This glycogen is stored in the liver and skeletal muscles. To break it down into glucose, calcium and another protein are needed. Once glycogen becomes glucose, the glucose splits into two molecules of pyruvic acid. This process, called *glycolysis*, releases energy.

In the process of glycolysis, oxygen is present. The next step is generally for the pyruvic acid to enter the mitochondria of the muscle cell. Here it is broken down, or *catabolized*, into carbon dioxide and water. This is an *aerobic* process (requiring oxygen to occur), and the entire metabolic process is called **cellular respiration**. This catabolism of pyruvic acid also yields energy for the contraction of the muscle fiber.

When there is not enough oxygen present to fully catabolize the pyruvic acid, most of it is converted to lactic acid. This can diffuse into the blood, releasing energy. Because this process occurs in the absence of oxygen, it is called *anaerobic*. This system is called the *glycogen–lactic acid system*.

For example, a hundred-meter dash would be the limit of the energy from the skeletal muscle source (fifteen seconds). That run is quadrupled to a four-hundred meter dash via the glycogen–lactic acid system (thirty to forty seconds). To sustain running a marathon, the aerobic system is up for the task—if there is adequate oxygen and nutrients.

The Nervous System

The nervous is headquarters and its cells are the cell managers. The system is made up of the brain, spinal cord, and nerves. Along with the endocrine system (which will be discussed soon), the nervous system controls and integrates body functions. Together, these two systems hold the homeostasis in your body.

In this communications network, the nerve tissues first sense internal and external changes, assess and interpret the changes, and then respond as needed. These changes could be temperature, pressure, heat, or light. The brain and spinal cord make up the *central nervous system (CNS)*, where all body sensations are processed. The cell managers in this system are responsible for rapid communications between cells and between organs. They accomplish this task by producing **neurotransmitters**, which activate and sustain nerve impulses. These electrical impulses can be sent from the CNS to any part of the body via the communications network of nerves.

Catecholamine neurotransmitters are the chemical substances present in brain cells which, when released, transmit signals to other cells in the brain or to muscle cells or secretory cells outside the brain. For the nervous system to function properly, sufficient amounts of neurotransmitters—such as dopamine, and norepinephrine and epinephrine—must be released into the synapses of the cells. They are made from amino acids, which we get from eating foods containing protein.

Neuropathy, a common complication of diabetes, affects nerve function in a variety of ways. It both interferes with nerve function and alters the message, resulting in a range of sensations. For some people the condition results in numbness. For others it can be felt as tingling, itching, or pain. Symptoms can be intermittent and can manifest in any part of the body, although the feet and legs are the most common sites. Neuropathy is caused by long-term high blood sugar levels, which change glucose into fructose and then into sorbitol. Once converted, this sugar cannot change back, so the nerve tissues cannot carry out their normal metabolism. This is called the *sorbitol pathway*.

Special Senses

Sensory cell workers bring vital information to headquarters about the environment in and around the factory. Their job is more specific than that of the general senses, even though the receptive and transmitting cells are neurons. Environmental changes are detected through the organs of smell, taste, touch, sight, hearing, equilibrium, and pheromones. Because diabetes has little effect on hearing, equilibrium, and pheromones, those senses are not discussed here.

The olfactory sensations (smell) are concentrated primarily in the nose and brain. For a smell to be detected, it must be in a gaseous state. It must also be water and fat soluble in order to pass through the membrane doors of the nostrils. Olfactory cell workers are alerted to odors through nerve endings in olfactory hairs. The impulse is sent along olfactory nerves to the olfactory bulb and along the olfactory tract to the cerebral cortex in the brain. There it is interpreted as one of more than fifty primal scents.

Approximately two thousand taste buds are employed in the sensation of taste, or gustatory senses. At the tip and sides of the tongue are fungiform papillae, taste buds that detect sweet, salt, and sour (although sweet taste is most concentrated at the tip and sour at the sides). Filliform papillae cover the front two-thirds of the tongue. They rarely contain taste buds. The large, round bumps that form a V at the back of the tongue are called circumvallate papillae. This area picks up bitter tastes before they enter the digestive tract. There are also some taste buds on the soft palate and in the throat.

The taste buds send the message to the brain that food is coming into the digestive system. The brain then sends out orders to release hormones and digestive enzymes along the digestive tract. Taste and smell work so closely together that a barrier to smell, such as a cold or allergy, severely alters the taste of food.

The eyeball is like the tip of an iceberg: only one-sixth of the structure is visible from the surface. Along with the optic nerve and supporting structures, this is the primary organ of the visual senses. Your eyeballs are highly protected in recessed areas of the bony skull. Eyebrows catch sweat and debris from above, and eyelids cover and lubricate your eyes.

In addition, an outer coat called a *fibrous tunic* covers the eyeball. On the outer, visible portion of the eye, this tunic is called the *sclera*. This "white of the eye" surrounds the *iris*, or colored portion of the eye. At the center of the iris is the *pupil*, which opens and closes to allow optimal light through to the *lens*. The lens is clear and is made up of special proteins that function as enzymes to convert sugar for energy in the lens. The iris and lens are part of the middle layer of the eyeball, the *vascular tunic*. Blood vessels and specialized muscles that work to change the shape of the lens from near to far vision are also in this layer. The nervous or *retinal tunic* is the third and innermost layer of the eye. This area contains the receptors of visual information, the optic nerve, and the retinal vein and artery. The optic nerve takes the information to the brain from the photoreceptors, called *rods* and *cones*. Rods are responsible for vision in light and dark tones, while cones deal with color. Night blindness or the inability to see in low light is generally due to a vitamin A deficiency.

It is in this retinal tunic area, where light is received and sent to the brain for interpretation, that diabetes takes a toll. Within twenty years of onset, nine out of ten people with diabetes experience vascular changes in the retina. This *background retinopathy* is generally caused by the breakdown of the **capillaries** (tiny blood vessels) in this area. They become weakened, can no longer carry adequate oxygen, form balloonlike bulges, and may rupture. For most people, these changes remain constant and can even improve. But about one in five people will progress to the next stage, called *proliferative retinopathy*. Blindness can still be prevented at this stage (even though diabetes is one of the leading causes of blindness). Severe eye problems are more common in type 1 diabetes and for people dependent on insulin. With proper nutrition and management of blood sugar levels, most people with diabetes can maintain or improve their condition. It is also critical to monitor and maintain blood pressure, since **hypertension** (high blood pressure) can cause retinopathy. Smoking adds an additional high risk to the list.

The Endocrine System

The cell managers assigned to the endocrine system coordinate with the nervous system to regulate the metabolic functions of the body. Together they form a highly coordinated network, stimulating and inhibiting each other's actions and reactions. They also have some distinct differences. Instead of sending messages to a specific part of the body via electrical impulses, the endocrine system moves information as chemicals called **hormones** through the bloodstream. This allows the endocrine cell managers to talk to any part of the body factory. Unlike the nervous system, which delivers messages rapidly, the endocrine system's chemical messengers can take their time and broadcast their information longer.

Hormones are delivered into the body factory through *endocrine glands*. Unlike *exocrine glands* (which squirt their substances into a duct that carries the secretions to their destination), endocrine glands deliver their product into the bloodstream via small capillary avenues. The endocrine system includes the pituitary, thyroid, parathyroid, pineal, adrenal, and thymus glands. Endocrine tissues also include the ovaries and testes, placenta, pancreas, kidneys, stomach, small intestine, heart, and skin.

The endocrine system sends a variety of messages to maintain balance and keep the factory running smoothly. Hormones tell the body when and how to grow. They receive the signals when the body is in an emergency, such as starvation, stress, infection, or temperature extremes, and they tell the appropriate departments how to respond. This system also helps the factory reproduce itself.

Since the **pancreas** is the organ responsible for blood sugar regulation, it is important to understand its relationship to diabetes. This organ is both an endocrine and an exocrine gland. In the endocrine portion there are three types of cells, situated in clusters called **islets of Langerhans**. The *alpha cells* secrete *glucagon* to raise blood sugar levels, the *beta cells* secrete insulin to lower blood sugar levels, and the *delta cells* secrete growth hormone inhibitor, or somatostatin, which inhibits the secretion of both insulin and glucagon.

The hormone glucagon increases blood sugar levels by telling the liver to convert more glycogen into glucose (a process called *glycogenolysis*). Amino acids, glycerol, and lactic acid are also directed to change into glucose (through *gluconeogenesis*). The liver then sends glucose into the bloodstream to raise blood sugar levels. At a certain level, the chemical sensors that told the glucagon to stimulate the liver turn off. If they fail to do so and the alpha cells keep sending out glucagon, high blood sugar can result.

The other side of the blood sugar equation is **insulin**. This hormone carries the blood sugar into the cells for energy. Insulin is the key that opens the cell door to let the sugar in. Insulin converts glucose into glycogen as well as into FAS (**fatty acids**). Insulin is also involved in the breakdown of proteins. Like glucagon, insulin takes its cue from the amount of sugar in the bloodstream. However, insulin production and release can be affected by an increase in amino acids and other hormones. Insulin can also be prevented from taking the glucose energy into the cell by a variety of defects at the molecular level. When deficiency or absence occurs and blood sugar levels are not controlled by insulin production, *diabetes mellitus* results.

When the alarms go off in the factory, they ring in the *adrenal glands*. This is called the "fight or flight" response. The adrenal medulla hormones secreted in stressful situations are epinephrine and norepinephrine. They increase blood pressure by increasing the heart rate and constricting the blood vessels. Breathing becomes more rapid, digestion decreases, and muscles contract faster because blood sugar levels increase with heightened cellular metabolism. Hyperglycemia occurs. This same response can be triggered by the opposite condition, hypoglycemia.

The Circulatory System

Every large and intricate factory must have a transport system designed to move products quickly from one area to another. For your body factory to function, oxygen must be picked up in one place, nutrients in another, and hormones from still other locations. These must be moved on and prepared to leave the body or used by the cells for energy. The system that facilitates that movement is called the *circulatory system*. The *cardiovascular system* is that part of the circulatory system that contains the heart, blood vessels, and blood. To protect the body from disease, the circulatory system also has a *lymphatic system*.

THE CARDIOVASCULAR SYSTEM

The structures of the cardiovascular system are a vast network of vessels and routes attached to a strong pump. The pump— your heart—is at the center of the system. **Arteries** carry blood filled with oxygen away from the heart to be taken to the cells via the capillaries. Here the oxygen trades places with carbon dioxide waste, which is sent back to the heart through the **veins**.

In order to send blood and take it way from remote places like a toe, the heart pump must be very strong and flexible. Muscle is the tissue for the job, pumping and pushing oxygen-depleted blood from the cells to the lungs to be cleaned of carbon dioxide waste. Renewed with oxygen, the blood returns to the heart and is taken back to the cells via the arteries.

The blood that is carried on this journey through the factory has both liquid and solid parts. The blood you see is sticky, warm, and red. The liquid plasma alone is straw-colored and carries important dissolved substances. Water makes up the largest portion of the plasma and is the solvent for proteins, wastes, nutrients, enzymes, salts and other **electrolytes**, gases, vitamins, minerals, blood sugar (glucose), and hormones such as insulin.

The solid parts of blood are the suspended cells. Red cells contain hemoglobin and are responsible for oxygen transport. The immune system has white cells (the good guys), which surround and attack intruders. To make sure your blood stays inside the factory and does not leak out, **platelets** are assigned to clot blood.

THE LYMPHATIC SYSTEM AND IMMUNITY

The cardiovascular system alone is not equipped to eliminate disease entering the bloodstream. Therefore, the lymphatic system polices the transport system and rids the body of unwanted intruders. This system includes lymphatic vessels, lymph nodes, lymph, tonsils, the thymus, and the spleen. Lymphatic tissue is also found in connective tissues of the gastrointestinal, urinary, respiratory, and reproductive tracts. In fact, it is found in the connective tissues of nearly every organ in the body. Even bone marrow plays a role in the production of lymphocytes, cells of the immune system.

These lymphocytes are programmed to detect troublemakers in the factory. The round lymph nodes are the places where they are taken for questioning. When a large enough group is in for examination, the lymph node enlarges and can be felt easily (especially on the neck, in the armpit, or in the groin). Sometimes the lymphocytes called T cells take out the intruders on their own with a special substance. Other times, B cells go undercover as plasma cells and secrete antibodies at the "bad guys." After the intruders are destroyed by *macrophages*, they are ushered out of the factory through the transport system. Macrophages are cell workers that are programmed to devour the enemy.

Besides the high-profile police work, the lymphatic system also transports fats and fluids. Because this transport system operates around the cardiovascular system, lymph picks up liquid that has escaped from blood and takes it back to the tissues.

The Respiratory System

All of the cell workers in the factory must have a constant supply of oxygen in order to use the energy from nutrients. At the same time, they must get rid of the carbon dioxide waste. The respiratory system networks with the circulatory system to accomplish this vital task. The first brings in and exchanges the gases, while the second transports them to the right departments in the factory.

The structures of the respiratory system include the nose, pharynx (throat), larynx, trachea, bronchi, and lungs. *Pulmonary ventilation*, or breathing, is the process of drawing fresh air from outside the factory into the lungs and sending out the old, stale air. That air is taken in through the nose, filtered by small hairs and warmed by body heat, and then drawn into the pharynx, over the larynx (site of the vocal cords), and into the trachea. C-shaped rings of cartilage make the trachea stiff yet flexible.

The trachea branches in the chest into two pathways at its base. This is the start of the *bronchi*, one side leading to the right lung and the other to the left lung. As the bronchi become smaller in diameter but larger in number, they are called *bronchioles* and then *alveoli* (air sacs). The alveolar sacs resemble tiny pouches that expand and contract with breathing. Here they give over their oxygen to the red cells in the capillaries lying directly under a thin membrane. The exchange of gases between the lungs and blood is called *external respiration*. This oxygen-rich blood is taken from the lungs to the heart and distributed through the arteries to the tissues. This stage is called *internal respiration*.

The left lung is divided into both a *superior* and an *inferior lobe*; the right lung also contains a *middle lobe*. In between the two lungs, in the *mediastinal surface*, lie the heart and aorta, the esophagus, trachea, nerves, lymphatic vessels, and bronchi. The heart sits in the cardiac notch of the left lung. These structures are all held together by connective tissue and a *pleural membrane*. A second pleural membrane lies on top of the lungs. The division between the lungs and abdominal cavity is called the *diaphragm*. It separates the upper body from the lower abdominal region and consists of strong muscle tissue that contracts and relaxes with the inspiration and expiration of the breath.

The Digestive System

The digestive system employs the food processors, the transportation crews, and the toxic waste engineers. The system functions around a long tube, the gastrointestinal (GI) tract (also called the **alimentary canal**) which extends from the mouth to the anus. It includes such organs as the *liver*, the *endocrine glands*, and the *pancreas*. The functions include mastication (chewing) of food; transportation of ingested substances; secretion of acid, mucus, digestive enzymes, and bile; digestion of food; and storage and excretion of waste products.

The digestive processes start in the *mouth*, where chewing mixes food with saliva, mucus, and the digestive enzyme ptyalin (salivary amylase), which begins to break down carbohydrates. Once food is softened in the mouth, it drops down the *esophagus* into the *stomach*. There, hydrochloric acid, intrinsic factor, the inactive protease pepsinogen, gastric lipase, mucus, and the hormone gastrin are released into the food. The stomach muscles roll the food around, mixing it with the digestive juices, but only a few fat-soluble substances and weak acids such as alcohol and aspirin are absorbed into the bloodstream.

Once the food is sufficiently softened and broken down, it is referred to as *chyme* and released by the gatekeeper known as the *pyloric sphincter* into the *small intestine*, where the bulk of the absorption and transportation take place. The small intestine consists of the *duodenum*, the *jejunum*, and the *ileum*. Just past the pyloric sphincter are the Brunner's glands, which secrete the mucus needed by the *duodenal tissue lining* as protection from the chyme's acidity.

Here the real action begins. The *liver* releases bile into the intestines, where it mixes with protein, carbohydrate, and fats and breaks them down to be absorbed. Bile is also responsible for termination and detoxification of hormones, **toxins**, and drugs. The pancreas produces enzymes such as pancreatic lipase, cholesterol esterase, pancreatic amylase, ribonuclease, deoxyribonuclease, carboxypolypeptidase, trypsin, chymotrypsin, and insulin and glucagon, the hormones that regulate blood sugar.

As the peristaltic waves of the intestines move the food along the intestinal tubing, the chyme is exposed to many digestive secretions; each acts on different aspects of the food. Each segment of the intestines secretes different enzymes and absorbs different nutrients. The small intestine secretes enzymes such as enterokinase, and the specialized epithelial cells secrete several peptidases, sucrase, lactase, alpha-dextrinase, maltase, amylase, and small quantities of enteric lipase.

By the time the bolus of final products reaches the *ileocecal valve*, most of the macronutrients have already been absorbed. The valve allows this material to pass from the small intestine into the *large intestine*, where electrolytes and water are absorbed. In the journey up the *ascending colon*, through the *transverse colon*, and down the *descending colon* to the *rectum*, a critical part of the digestive process takes place. In the large intestine are trillions of living organisms known as the microflora. These healthful bacteria colonize in the gut, where they aid in the final stages of digestion and actually make some vitamins. The remaining materials are indigestible fiber and toxic waste products, which are propelled by contractions of the colon and the rectum and expelled through the *anal sphincter*.

> A considerable body of scientific data suggests a positive relationship between vegetarian meal plans and risk reduction for several chronic degenerative diseases and conditions, including obesity, coronary artery disease, hypertension, diabetes, and some types of cancer.
>
> ADA *Reports*, "Position of the American Diabetes Association: Vegetarian Diets."

ORGANS OF THE DIGESTIVE SYSTEM

As we discussed, the pancreas is the organ that produces insulin. When the beta cells in the islets of Langerhans are healthy, they produce insulin in response to a rise in blood sugar levels. The higher the blood sugar and the more rapid the rise, the more insulin is released to compensate. This keeps the blood sugar from skyrocketing. Insulin removes the potentially damaging excess sugar from the bloodstream and takes it to the liver and muscle tissue if needed or to fat cells for storage.

When the pancreas turns on the insulin production and distribution, the adrenal glands must produce adrenaline to turn off the process. The adrenaline keeps blood sugar from plummeting below normal fasting levels, a condition called **hyperinsulinism**. This excess of insulin interferes with production of glucagon and growth hormones. This in turn affects lean body mass, muscle building, and body (or cell) repair.

The Urinary System

The urinary system employs the sanitary engineers of the factory. Their job is to clean the waste from the bloodstream transport system. They collect the waste from all the body organs, filtering, cleaning, and eliminating it in the kidneys, ureters, bladder, and urethra. Approximately seventeen hundred liters of blood are cleaned to produce a single liter of urine concentrate in a day.

The *kidneys* filter the blood through a vast network of capillaries and form the urine. These organs are essential to maintaining homeostasis through the control of blood volume and composition. They play a role in making red blood cells, controlling the acid–base balance of blood, regulating blood pressure, and activating vitamin D. As the urine is collected in the kidneys, it is sent through the tubular structure of the *ureters* to the *bladder*. The bladder is hollow and made mostly of muscular tissue so it can expand as it fills to store the urine. When it reaches a certain level of fullness, it sends the brain a signal to empty it through the *urethra* and out. By maintaining and storing fluids, the kidneys are essential to the balance of water, electrolytes, and acid in the body.

In long-term diabetes, the walls that form the capillaries in the kidneys tend to thicken and become more porous. The proteins they are supposed to concentrate and store spill into the urine instead. This can produce uremia as toxic levels of nitrogen waste products from the urine accumulate in the blood. The extreme level of toxicity leads to kidney failure and can be treated only by dialysis or a kidney transplant. Diabetics are prone to bladder infections and high blood pressure, both of which can lead to kidney complications. Proper maintenance and strict control of blood sugar can prevent and sometimes reverse certain kidney damage.

Blood: The Transportation System for Nutrients

Blood is like a freeway on which the village transports the goods to the cells and tissues of the body. High-traffic times are after meals, when fats, proteins, and sugars are all going to their respective tissues.

High blood sugar results when too much sugar is in the bloodstream. You can think of insulin as a cab taking the sugar to the correct houses (cells). Chromium is the key to getting in. Chromium opens the passage into the cell, which allows the insulin and sugar to enter, thus providing energy. Without chromium, insulin is very inefficient in delivering sugar out of the bloodstream and into the cells, which results in higher blood sugar levels. Once all the sugar has found a home, then blood sugar levels drop and the freeway runs smoothly again.

Anatomy and Physiology and the "Little People"

I want to share a story from our local newspaper here in Seattle, Washington. The author is Jennifer James, a cultural anthropologist, who has a weekly column in the *Seattle Times*. This is a wonderful way for us all to think about our bodies and about taking care of our "little people" who take such good care of us. If you're like me, you'll remember the little people and their work long after you have forgotten an anatomy lesson.

I got the idea when I was ten, while watching a film in school. It was called "Hemo the Magnificent," and it was about the bloodstream. I felt intense during this film, realizing my body was full of red-cell guys swimming downstream, white-cell guys struggling upstream, and lots of workers opening and closing the valves. I decided it was important to treat all the corpuscles with respect.

I kept this idea about all my cells being tiny people with me until, as an adult, I saw Woody Allen's *Everything You Ever Wanted to Know About Sex . . . But Were Afraid to Ask*.

My ideas about the little people have multiplied since Allen's movie. I started to watch what I ate because the stomach people had such a messy job. They had to navigate their kayaks around all the stuff, particularly fat globs, and add just the right amount of acid. I didn't want them in a toxic environment so I gave up bacon cheeseburgers.

I could imagine them complaining about their working conditions: "Can you believe she's eating another dessert? Last week I got my paddle stuck in a Twinkie." It hurt me to hear them fussing.

The air movers in the lungs are usually mellow. They prefer to wear pink sweatshirts and puff about endlessly. But when I am in a smoky environment, I can sense that their soft shirts are turning hard and brown and they are looking at themselves, upset. They have long conversations late at night trying to decide how to wash everything.

The brain is a large round room with a dome and a fireplace in the middle. The cells are arranged on cots or chairs in circles around the fire. They muse a lot, read a lot; it is generally quiet. There are occasional well-mannered arguments among friends. A few of the younger ones cause trouble with radical thoughts, but it is becoming more of an old girls' club than a free-for-all.

When I am sad I can see them all lying around moping. They let the fire go out, close the windows so it is dark, and stop reading or talking. I get the message that they need exercise, but no one will move. It doesn't happen much anymore because the wisdom cells, the ones in the long white robes, give them a gentle lecture, and then they all relight the fire and have tea.

Everyone loves massage. All the tiny cell people from the top to bottom stretch out, serene smiles on their faces, waiting for their turn. If you miss one, it will complain until enough signals are sent to command attention. Promises are made during massages; contracts are signed. Each team vows to take better care of each other. They have sing-alongs and humming contests.

I've been much happier since I accepted the theory of the little people. I listen to them carefully. Mine are getting louder and many of them have started wearing plastic pants. At one of the last general meetings they demanded a shorter workweek and loose shoes. Right now the stomach cells are on their tiny pogo sticks wanting to go out.

So I'm going for a walk in the sunshine. I'm willing to please all of them. They take care of me, so I plan to give them anything they want.

Tune into your body, listen to those tiny voices, take better care of yourself, and sooner or later you will hear them cheer.

3

The Glycemic Index

$\mathcal{N}$ow that we have looked at anatomy and physiology and how our bodies absorb food, let's look at blood sugar (glucose) levels and what influences them. The **glycemic index** is a way to categorize foods depending on how they affect blood sugar levels. On a scale of one hundred, the index ranges from about ten for soybeans to eighty for jelly beans. The idea is to avoid foods that are high on the index, since they have a great potential to raise blood sugar levels. We recommend that your meal plan emphasize foods that are below forty on the glycemic index. The table beginning on page 32 provides the glycemic indexes of various foods.

Several factors influence a food's effect on postprandial (after a meal) blood sugar. **Fiber** content has a profound effect on the digestion time of food. High-fiber foods take longer to digest, so they release smaller amounts of glucose into the bloodstream over a longer period of time. This results in a lower glycemic response. Factors that tend to increase the glycemic factor of foods are the level of processing and refining, natural sugar, added sugars, and their carbohydrate, fat, and protein content.

How Mixing Foods Affects the Glycemic Response

When foods that are high on the glycemic index (such as ice cream) are eaten with foods that are low on the index (such as beans), the entire meal mixes in the stomach and has a new glycemic index. Now the sugars in the ice cream will not raise blood sugar levels as dramatically as if it were eaten alone. The entire meal will have a slower rate of absorption, which allows for better blood sugar control.

Legumes and the Glycemic Index

Legumes such as beans, peas, and lentils have a very flat glycemic response. This is especially true of soybeans, which are rich in the gel-forming soluble fibers and enzyme inhibitors. Enzyme inhibitors occur naturally in food and slow down its digestion and absorption in the small intestine.

A meal plan rich in legumes is high in both carbohydrates and fiber. Many patients on a high-leguminous meal plan can reduce the amount of insulin they are taking; some on lower doses can eventually eliminate it. (Anderson and Ward 1979) It appears that a high-fiber meal plan enhances the cell receptivity to insulin by increasing receptor sites on the monocyte cells. (Anderson 1979) This lowers fasting and postprandial plasma glucose as well as insulin requirements. Viscous soluble fibers such as guar and pectin help to flatten the glycemic response in both normal and diabetic individuals. This effect may be due to the fiber's ability to slow the rate at which the digestive enzymes break down food for absorption in the intestines.

The Glycemic Index

Baked Products	Value
whole-meal rye	41
pita bread, white	57
hamburger bun	61
white bagel	72
French baguette	95

Breakfast Cereals	Value
All-Bran	30
Muesli	43
Bran Chex	58

Grape-Nuts	67
Cheerios	74
Grape-Nuts Flakes	80
Cornflakes	80
Rice Krispies	82
Crispix	87

Whole Grains	Value
barley	22
pearled barley	29
brown rice	50
long-grain white rice	58
millet	71
instant rice	87

Dairy Foods	Value
whole milk	27
skim milk	32

Fruits	Value
cherries	22
plum	24
grapefruit	25
peach	28
banana, underripe	30
pear	33
apple	39
grapes	43
orange	43
banana, overripe	52
kiwi	52
orange juice	57
pawpaw	58
mango	60
pineapple	66
watermelon	72

Vegetables	Value
peanuts	14
sweet potato	54
beets	64
carrots	71
baked potato	85
instant potatoes	88
parsnips	97

Legumes	Value
soybeans	10
peas	22
red beans	26
kidney beans	27
lentils	29
butter beans	31
split peas	32
lima beans	32
chickpeas	33
black-eyed peas	42
pinto beans	45

Pasta	Value
spaghetti	41
macaroni	45
linguine	46
rice pasta	92

"The International Tables of Glycemic Index," *The American Journal of Clinical Nutrition* 1995; 62:87S–93S. The American Society of Clinical Nutrition.

4

Carbohydrates and the
Glycemic Index

$\mathcal{W}$hole foods are made of three basic macronutrients: carbo-hydrates (which all break down into sugar in the body), fat (an important source of cholesterol and triglycerides), and protein (which becomes sugar, enzymes, hormones, muscles, and other tissue). All three **macronutrients** are energy sources (calo-ries) that allow your body cells to function properly. All of the macronutrients enter the body in complex forms and are broken down through the metabolic processes of catabolism into their basic components.

Defining Carbohydrates

Carbohydrate is the primary nutrient in food that affects blood sugar (glucose) levels. Many factors affect foods' poten-tial for glycemic response, among them timing, quality, quan-tity, processing, nutrient and fiber content, and ratio compared to other foods eaten at the same time. **Simple carbohydrates** are simple sugars such as glucose molecules, which may be burned immediately for energy or brain activity. If the energy is not needed immediately, then the glucose is stored in the mus-cles as glycogen. After all of the storage space in the muscles gets filled, the excess glucose is converted into fat and stored in fat (adipose) cells.

It is important to be familiar with the different guises in which simple carbohydrates or sugars may hide, especially in processed foods. The only way to know what food products contain sugar is to read the labels and become familiar with the many names that mean sugar. This alphabetical list explains which sugars you can safely include in your meal plan and which to avoid.

- *Alcohol* can displace nutritive foods. Beer, wine, and spirits are simple carbohydrates. Alcohol has the potential to cause high blood sugar levels because it becomes sugar in the bloodstream within minutes. Minimize alcohol intake, and take it only with food.

- *Artificial sweeteners*, also known as synthetic sweeteners, are not whole foods. They are man-made products that have no nutritional value and cause many negative effects. Many of the synthetic sweeteners available today are also suspected of adding to blood sugar instability. See Chapter 19 for more information.

- **Complex carbohydrates** are also known as starches. Legumes, whole grains, and vegetables contain them. Complex carbohydrates should make up 50 percent of your daily meal plan.

- *Dextrose* is a form of glucose extracted from corn, sugar cane, and sugar beets. It should be avoided.

- *Disaccharides* are two monosaccharides linked together. This is a chemical name not generally used on food labels or in cookbooks. The word *saccharide* means sugar, and this term indicates simple sugars. Avoid these simple sugars.

- *Fructose* is sugar that is generally found in fruits, saps, honey, berries, and vegetables. It is the sweetest of the true sugars. Foods containing fructose that are high in fiber—such as apples, blueberries, and strawberries—can be eaten as part of a meal. However, refined forms of fructose, such as corn syrup should be avoided, since high concentrations will raise blood sugar and triglyceride levels. High-fructose corn syrup is found in soft drinks and candies. A monosaccharide, fructose is also known as fruit sugar or levulose.

Fructose can be absorbed through the intestinal wall directly into the bloodstream. When the blood circulates past the liver, the fructose is taken up into the liver cells, where enzymes rearrange the atoms to make compounds indistinguishable from those derived from glucose and sometimes to make glucose itself. Fructose does not need insulin to get into the cells. It has a somewhat greater tendency to be converted to fat than to glycogen (stored blood sugar in the liver), a tendency that contributes to high levels of fat in the blood. So people with elevated triglycerides should be aware that fructose may raise triglyceride levels.

- *Glucose* is the main sugar of our meal plans and metabolic energy. Both complex and simple carbohydrates are converted to glucose during metabolism. When food breaks down in your stomach and intestines into glucose, it travels the bloodstream ready for action. The brain and muscles use glucose as fuel. The excess is converted to glycogen, which is stored in the muscles or the liver.

  Glucose is known as blood sugar. Like most monosaccharides, it is absorbed rapidly into the bloodstream from the intestines and through the lining of the mouth. In cases of extreme hypoglycemia—such as insulin shock—when a quick supply of glucose is needed, it can be administered via the mouth. It will then be absorbed directly into the bloodstream. Check the fine print on food labels and you will find that glucose is hidden in a variety of processed foods, from ham and sausage to ketchup and breads.

- *Glycogen* is what glucose stored in the liver is converted to. Glycogen can then be used for brain fuel or energy or changed into protein if necessary.

- *Glycyrrhiza*, extracted from licorice root, is approved in the United States as a flavor enhancer. Regular use can raise blood pressure, so it is not recommended for those who have high blood pressure. Licorice root extracts are now available in liquid or powdered form. Licorice root has a distinct black licorice flavor and makes a delicious tea. It is a promising safe sweetener for people with diabetes. Licorice root is used medicinally for hypoglycemia, bronchitis, colitis, diverticulosis, gastritis, stress, colds, nausea, and inflammation. It cleanses the colon, promotes adrenal gland function, decreases muscle or skeletal spasms, and increases fluidity of mucus from the lungs and bronchial tubes.

- *Lactose* is milk sugar, which is made up of glucose and galactose. Because it is made of two sugars it is called a disaccharide. Lactose tastes slightly sweet. It is commonly used in the food industry as an additive to help keep moisture in foods. It is also used as a medical diuretic and laxative.
- *Licorice root.* See glycyrrhiza.
- *Levulose* is simply another name for granulated fructose.
- *Maltose* is the sugar present in germinating grain. Seeds naturally contain glucose that the seed uses as fuel as it sprouts into a plant. When the seed begins to sprout, an enzyme cleaves the chains of glucose units into pairs of glucose molecules, or maltose. Other enzymes break the maltose down further to glucose. This is why malt sugars made from sprouting plants have such a distinct malt flavor and why they are so sweet.
- *Monosaccharides* are single sugar units (*mono* means one, and *saccharide* means sugar). Glucose is an example of a monosaccharide.
- *Polysaccharides* are complex sugar units (*poly* means many, and *saccharide* means sugar). Polysaccharides are sugars found in complex carbohydrates.
- *Simple carbohydrates* are both mono- and disaccharides, also known as simple sugars. Table sugar (sucrose), honey maple syrup, fruit sugar (fructose), and corn syrup are simple carbohydrates.
- *Sucrose* is the chemical name for common table sugar. Commercially found as sugar-cane granules, powder, or sugar-

beet products, sucrose breaks down into glucose and fructose in the digestive tract. Aside from calories, sucrose provides little nutrition, and it can stimulate fat production in the body.

Various Kinds of Carbohydrates

As carbohydrates metabolize, they become indigestible and digestible fibers, as well as simple sugars. Almost all foods contain some carbohydrates. The trick is to know which carbohydrate foods release too much simple sugar and then to minimize their intake.

Polysaccharides from the stalks and leaves of vegetables and the outer coverings of seeds break down into *cellulose* and *hemicellulose*. They can be broken down further when bacterial action in the large intestines splits apart some of the glucose molecules from these polysaccharides. *Pectin*, *gums*, and *mucilages* come from plant secretions and seeds. They have an affinity for water and form bulk, which has the beneficial effect of slowing gastric emptying and stimulating the peristaltic action of the intestines. Seaweeds and algae are very beneficial food sources for blood sugar regulation as their end products are indigestible polysaccharides.

The partially digestible forms of polysaccharides come from foods such as Jerusalem artichokes, onions, garlic, and mushrooms, which release *fructose*, and legumes, which metabolize into *mannose*. *Mannose* is worth a mention as it is one of the sugars that our bodies have a hard time completely metabolizing and can cause gas.

Grains such as rice, wheat, and oats will break down to release *glucose*, which is simple sugar, into the bloodstream. It is thus important to eat grains in small quantities along with high-fiber foods, such as legumes, which will help slow the metabolism and release of glucose into the bloodstream.

Disaccharides and *oligosaccharides* are even simpler forms of carbohydrates. They are shorter carbon chains which break down quickly into sugars in the digestive tract. For example, sucrose is found in foods such as beet sugar, cane sugar, molasses, and maple syrup. These break down into glucose and fructose.

The *monosaccharides* are *glucose*—found in fruits, honey, and corn syrup—and *fructose*—found in fruits and honey. These simple forms of sugar are quickly absorbed into the bloodstream where they can stockpile. This causes high blood sugar levels until there is enough insulin—either released by the pancreas or injected—to take each of those molecules of simple sugar into cells.

Minimize your intake of all sweeteners such as honey, molasses, maple syrup, date sugar, and cane sugar (white and unrefined turbinado) and watch food labels for sugar which comes in many forms under terms such as *sucrose, fructose, maltose, glucose, mannitol, sorbitol, galactose, corn syrup*, and so on.

Quick-Acting Carbohydrates to Avoid

Check labels to avoid consuming much of these carbohydrates in processed foods.

fructose	levulose
maltose	corn syrup
lactose	high-fructose corn syrup
glucose	date sugar
galactose	turbinado sugar
monosaccharides	brown sugar
polysaccharides	confectioner's sugar
sucrose	invert sugar

Carbohydrate Metabolism

Carbohydrates must be broken down into their component monosaccharides before they can be absorbed. The glucose absorbed through the intestine immediately goes into the portal vein, which transports it to the liver and eventually the bloodstream. As a meal is digested, the amount of blood glucose rises. In response to the glucose in the blood, the islets of Langerhans in the pancreas secrete the hormone insulin into the blood. This means glucose and insulin reach the hungry cell at the same time. Glucose cannot enter a cell without insulin. Insulin is like a key that opens the cell door or receptor site. When not enough insulin is secreted, the cells can be surrounded by glucose but unable to use it since all their doors are locked. This is the dilemma in diabetes; some of the excess sugar is excreted in the urine and can be detected by a urine test.

Sometimes when insulin and glucose meet before a hungry cell, they find that there are few doors for the glucose to enter through. This results in **insulin resistance**, also referred to as a decrease in *insulin tolerance*.

When the glucose enters a cell, it has several options:

- If the cell is hungry, the glucose is used immediately to make energy.
- If the cell is not hungry, the glucose is changed by muscle and liver cells into glycogen for temporary storage.
- If the storage room for glycogen is filled up, the remaining glucose is changed into fat and stored in regular cells or in the fat-storage (adipose) cells.

The next time cells get hungry and no glucose is available from a meal, the glycogen stored in the muscles and liver is changed back into glucose and fed to them. When the glycogen is used up, fat is used to make glucose. This stimulates the appetite, causing you to eat more and make more glucose available. The process of making new glucose is called **gluconeogenesis** (*gluco* = sugar, *neo* = new, *genesis* = creation).

Fructose is also absorbed into the portal system. In the liver its atoms are rearranged to form glucose. The liver then releases the glucose as needed.

Natural Sweeteners

The following definitions will help you sort out the wide variety of sweeteners on the market today. Remember that even a sweetener that is natural and contains more vitamins and/or minerals than white refined sugar has the same potential to raise blood sugar levels and must be used sparingly.

- *Barley malt syrup* has a dark brown color, a thick and sticky texture (like molasses), and a rich malt flavor. It is generally used in baked goods and baked beans. Buy only 100 percent barley products; others contain corn malt syrup, which dilutes flavor and increases sugar content. Buy organic products when possible. Barley malt tends to be thick, so the lid may stick. If this happens, run hot water over the jar lid to help liquefy it.

- *Brown rice syrup* has an amber color and mild butterscotch flavor. It is not as sweet as white sugar and is best used in granolas, cookies, crisps, pies, and puddings. It tends to get hard and crisp and mixes well with other sweeteners. Organic products are available.

- *Brown sugar* is white table sugar with molasses added to it. Its brown coloration comes from a charcoal treatment that may introduce traces of **carcinogenic** impurities, resulting in a product that is actually more refined and possibly more harmful than white sugar.

- *Cane sugar*, unrefined and raw, contains trace nutrients such as chromium, manganese, cobalt, copper, zinc, and molybdenum. Filtering and leaching cane juice produces bleached white table sugar, stripped of all nutrients. Bleaching also adds a questionable element to the sugar. See turbinado sugar in this section for more information on unrefined cane sugar.

- *Corn syrup* is cornstarch made into sweet dextrose syrup. It is cheap to make and often used in commercial food products such as cakes, cookies, beverages, ice cream, and candy. It is also used on envelopes, stamps, sticking tapes, and in aspirin and many food products, including bacon, baking mixes, powders, beer, bourbon, breads, breakfast cereals, pastries, ketchup, cheeses, fish products, ginger ale, jellies, processed meats, peanut butter, canned peas, plastic food wraps, sherbet, whiskey, and American wines.

- *Date sugar* is a coarse granular product with a mahogany color produced from ground dehydrated dates. It does contain some folic acid. Whole-date puree is a superior sweetener. Purchase whole, pitted dates, puree them in the blender with water to the desired consistency, and add to baked goods. Date sugar is ideal for making chewy cookies. Dates contain considerable amounts of soluble and insoluble fiber. Always purchase unsulfured, organically grown dates.

- *Dried cane juice* is extracted from sugar cane and dried into amber granules that have a mild molasseslike flavor. Many pesticides and chemicals are used in the growing of sugar cane, so it is important to only use organic sugar-cane juice.

- *Fruit juice concentrate* is made from a variety of fruits, generally peach, pear, grape, or pineapple juice. It has a definite fruit taste and can be used in all baked goods. Fruit juice consists mainly of fructose. Although this sweetener is made from whole natural fruit, it is extracted from the fruit's natural fibers, which means that the fruit's sugars will be absorbed quickly into your bloodstream. Use fruit sweetener as sparingly as you would any other kind of sugar.

- *Honey* is made by bees from flower nectar. Since it is sweeter than white sugar, you can use less of it. Honey's color and flavor differ depending on the flowers from which it came. For example, clover honey tastes much differently from alfalfa honey. There are a few drawbacks to using honey as a sweetener. Children under the age of two years should never eat honey because it can transmit enough botulism to be very dangerous to them. Honey can also raise blood sugar levels, so it must be used sparingly.

- *Invert sugar* is a mix of half glucose and half fructose. It is sweeter than sucrose and therefore makes an ideal product for commercial use. It is used commercially but is not commonly available to consumers.

- *Malt extract* is extracted from barley that has been allowed to germinate, then heated, dried, and ground into a slightly sweet-flavored powder. It is often used as a commercial additive in foods such as vinegar, brewing beer, and distilled liquor, but it is rarely available to consumers.

- *Maltodextrin* is obtained by the hydrolysis of starch. A combination of maltol and dextrin, it is used as a flavor enhancer, particularly in chocolates and candies. This sugar alcohol is found in many plants but is mostly prepared from seaweed. It does contain calories and carbohydrates but has a lower glycemic effect, as it is more slowly absorbed and metabolized to fructose than sucrose is. The Food and Drug Administration (FDA) is studying it because it can cause gastrointestinal disturbances such as flatulence and diarrhea and may worsen kidney disease. It's best to avoid maltodextrin until further studies are done.

- *Mannitol* is a white, crystalline, odorless powder that has half the calories of, and is two-thirds as sweet as, table sugar. Prepared from seaweed, this carbohydrate is used in food products and cosmetics. It is under study by the FDA because it can cause gastrointestinal disturbances and diarrhea. It is used as a baby laxative to soften the stools. People with kidney disease are advised to avoid this product.

- *Maple sugar* is granulated (dehydrated) maple syrup. It is light brown in color and has that telltale maple flavor. Try to purchase organic products whenever possible. Store in an airtight container and sift before using.

- *Maple syrup* is dark brown with maple flavor. Some syrups are made mostly of processed refined white table sugar or corn syrup with a small quantity of maple; their flavor is inferior to the real thing. Then there are the maple syrups flavored with synthetic sweeteners, which taste like the chemicals they are made from. Pure maple syrup comes from the sap of maple trees and is rich in potassium and calcium. Buy only pure U.S. organic syrup, because many producers still use illegal formaldehyde pellets and other additives in processing.

- *Molasses* is a by-product of granulated table sugar production. Blackstrap molasses is the liquid that remains after all the sucrose crystals are removed from sugar cane. It contains the cane's original minerals. There are several different varieties. New Orleans molasses is made from the juice of young Louisiana-grown sugar canes. It is classified as sulfured because it is clarified using sulfur dioxide. Product packaging specifies sulfured or unsulfured. Unsulfured, or Barbados, molasses is mild and sweet in flavor. Made from the whole juice of mature East Indian cane, it is free from sulfur but has considerably reduced mineral content. Dried molasses is a blend of corn syrup, wheat starch, soy flour, and preservatives.

- *Sorbitol* is a sugar alcohol that is half as sweet as table sugar. This polyalcohol is found naturally in a variety of plants and is also produced commercially from monosaccharides. It has a lower glycemic effect because of its slow absorption and metabolism to fructose, but it can cause diarrhea and digestive problems.

- *Stevia* is derived from the leaf of a berry plant native to South America. Stevioside is a natural, low-calorie sweetener that has been harvested for centuries. The stevia herb, which is grown in Paraguay, is not as strong as the stevia leaf from China. Stevia can be used to sweeten drinks,

baked goods, and cereals, among other foods. It is the safest
known sweetener for diabetics to use. It is available in powder or liquid form.

- *Sugar alcohols* have a calorie count similar to that of table
  sugar and are derived commercially from dextrose and glucose. Once broken down by the digestive system, sugar
  alcohols act like all other forms of sugar. See also sorbitol
  in this section.

- *Turbinado sugar* is a steam-cleaned version of raw sugar that
  retains a fraction of its dark, sticky molasses syrup and
  therefore a fraction of its original minerals. It is known as
  Demerara sugar when it comes from the Demerara region
  of Guyana.

Alternative Sweeteners

There are few safe, flavorful, no-calorie, natural alternative
sweeteners today. Stevia is now available through mail-order
sources (see Resources in the Appendix) in liquid and powdered
form to be used for sweetening and cooking. Licorice-root
extract can also be used as a sweetener.

The key to success with sugar in the meal plan is in the quantity, quality, and timing. A maximum of 5 percent of total carbohydrates is suggested as an acceptable intake per day. For
example, in a 1,800-**calorie** meal plan with 50 percent (or
900 calories) as carbohydrate, 5 percent equals 45 calories
(11.2 grams of carbohydrate). One teaspoon of table sugar contains 16 calories (4 grams of carbohydrate). Total sugar intake
for the day for this person would be approximately 3 teaspoons
of sugar. Consume sugar only with meals (ideally whole fresh
foods) so that the sugar mixes with the fiber-containing foods
and gets absorbed slowly. Sugar is a natural part of foods such
as beets, carrots, apples, and strawberries, and this is the best
type of sugar to eat.

Americans consume so much sugar that it may take some
awareness training to start noticing how much sugar is currently

in your diet. The average intake of sucrose in the United States has been estimated at 41 grams. That's a quarter cup of sugar a day.

Natural sugars are "nutritive" and contain calories, but *natural* does not necessarily mean they are unrefined or "nutritious." Many natural sweeteners are highly processed and add little more than blood sugar–raising calories to the diet.

Added sugars make up a substantial amount of many food products. Some may surprise you. They include breads, candies, canned goods, cereals, condiments, frozen dinners, fruit drinks, ketchup, soft drinks, soups, spaghetti sauces, and even yogurts.

Types of Carbohydrate Foods

Learn how carbohydrates affect blood sugar and you can harness the healthful energy that they provide. First, take control of your blood glucose levels by eating the same amount of carbohydrate at each meal and the same amount at each snack.

Carbohydrate counting has become popular because it allows people with diabetes more freedom in food choices. But all carbohydrates are not created equal. There is a tremendous difference in overall health effects of different carbohydrates. For example, 12 grams of carbohydrate in the form of a slice of white bread will have a spiking effect on blood sugar. Compare that to 12 grams of pinto beans, which metabolize more slowly and help to control blood sugar.

Grains, legumes, vegetables, and fruit are all good carbohydrate sources. Dairy foods, generally speaking, are not. Consider the total amount of both simple and complex carbohydrates in your meal plan. The fiber, vitamin, mineral, and **phytochemical** contents of carbohydrates all change the way they affect blood sugar. Whole-grain cereals that are rich in complex carbohydrates metabolize more slowly than others. Whole grains have an intact germ, which contains beneficial fat-soluble vitamins.

Dairy Foods

Because dairy foods are high in fat (including saturated fat and cholesterol), contain no fiber, are a common allergenic food group, displace more nutrient-dense foods, and may contain bovine growth hormone, their consumption should be reduced. However yogurt, small quantities of cheese, and low-fat or non-fat milk may be used sparingly.

Grains

Whole, unrefined grains such as barely, slow-cooking oats, and rye have a safe glycemic range, between thirty and fifty. They also contain the mineral chromium, which regulates blood sugar. (Boyle et al. 1977) The value of chromium in blood sugar regulation is well established. (Haylock 1983, Mertz 1993, Freund 1979) Processed foods are inherently deficient in chromium—a deficiency that may contribute to the prevalence of glucose intolerance in the United States and Western Europe.

DEFINING GRAINS

Grains in their whole, uncut, unground form are called berries. These berries can be cooked whole and eaten like hot cereal. They can also be used to accompany vegetables and legumes, as you would use rice. Grains that test higher in the glycemic index—such as rice (puffed, instant, or white), millet, and fast-cooking oats—should be avoided. The list on the opposite page covers grains that are good for you:

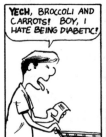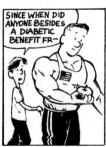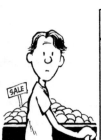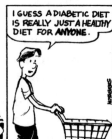

- *Amaranth* grain and flour products provide an alternative to wheat.
- *Barley* is a whole grain that is very high in chromium, about 5.69 micrograms per gram.
- *Corn* can be used in corn tortillas, corn bread, and cornmeal.
- *Kamut* is available in cereals, flour crackers, and whole berries.
- *Oats* can be eaten as oatmeal, oat-bran cereal, and steel-cut oats.
- *Quinoa* can be cooked for a breakfast cereal or a rice alternative in savory dishes.
- *Brown rice* products include rice bread, rice noodles, rice cereals, rice milk, and mochi.
- *Rye* crackers, which contain only rye flours, salt, and water, are available. There are also 100 percent rye breads available. Cereals containing rye grain can be found in health-food stores and specialty markets.
- *Spelt* flour is high in gluten and makes wonderful bread. Spelt cereals, crackers, and breads are now available.
- *Teff* grains cooked with broth make a savory side dish.
- *Whole-wheat* bagels, bread, cereals, chapati, crusts, pancakes, pasta, pretzels, rolls, tortillas, and waffles are available.

A diabetic whole-plant-foods meal plan should contain whole-grain foods that are high in fiber, high in complex carbohydrates, and rich in chromium, biotin, pyridoxine, copper, manganese, magnesium, zinc, phosphorus, and potassium. All of these improve blood glucose tolerance.

The goal of this program is to reduce the risk of diabetic complications by controlling blood sugar, cholesterol, triglycerides, and blood pressure. Conveniently, this whole-foods meal plan is the healthiest way to eat for everyone. Whole foods are foods that are as unprocessed and unadulterated as possible. They are in their whole, natural form, without added preservatives and colorings.

The refining process of removing the germ and bran from grains renders them nutritionally inferior to whole, unrefined foods. Refining removes much of the vitamins, minerals, and fiber from the original whole food. For example, when whole-wheat flour is processed, it loses its vitamin- and mineral-containing germ and its fiber-containing bran component. The endosperm is then bleached and used to make white flour.

Avoid packaged and processed foods. Whole grains are complex carbohydrates but white flour, white bread, pasta, and pastries are not. Refined carbohydrate products also often contain bleaches, preservatives, colorings, and other chemicals that reduce their quality.

Grains to Avoid

The following grains are too high on the glycemic index to be healthful for those with diabetes.

couscous	millet
instant rice	white rice

Simple carbohydrates are monosaccharides and disaccharides such as lactose (milk sugar), sucrose (cane sugar), and fructose (fruit sugar). The most widely used sweeteners—white table sugar, corn syrup, and honey—are all made of sucrose and fructose. They should be consumed sparingly and only with a meal. Simple sugar is quickly metabolized and absorbed, causing a rise in blood sugar. But simple sugars will be absorbed more slowly if you eat them with high-fiber foods. The sugars mix with the other foods in the stomach, which slows their breakdown and absorption, reducing the overall glycemic index of the stomach's contents.

Many foods containing sugar are known as "empty calorie" foods. This slang nutrition term refers to a food that has a lot of calories but adds few nutrients to the meal plan. Candy, pastries, and sodas are empty calorie foods. If you want to have a sugary food, substitute it in a small amount for a carbohydrate choice in your meal plan. Simple sugar should be limited to 5 percent or less of total carbohydrate calories. Choose homemade, whole-grain cookies sweetened with stevia or soy-based desserts. Combine foods within the same meal to stay between 50 and 80 on the glycemic index as much as possible. Eating beans and a small piece of candy, for example, is fine as long as you stay in this range. This is also why sweets should be eaten with a meal.

Grains and the Little People

The little people appreciate a hearty meal of whole grains, such as a bowl of oatmeal, far more than a bowl of refined carbohydrate, such as cornflakes. The oatmeal breaks down slowly, releasing smaller quantities of sugar into the bloodstream at a time. The little nutrient transportation guys who are responsible for getting that sugar to the cells have a much easier time when they are not overloaded with work. Slow release of sugar allows them to organize the chromium and insulin they will need for transporting the sugar into the cell as well as to find cells that need immediate energy or storage places in the liver or muscle tissue. By contrast, refined carbohydrates break down so quickly that the bloodstream winds up loaded with vast amounts of sugar (high blood glucose level), and all the transportation workers become exhausted.

To summarize, carbohydrates are broken down in the digestive system into the most highly available form of simple sugars. The more slowly this process takes place, the longer your blood sugar will remain at a safe level. Whole grains and legumes are complex carbohydrates and therefore good choices for the daily meal plan. Simple sugars are found in a wide range of food products, so it's essential to learn to read food labels. (See Chapter 16 for an analysis of nutrition labels.) Be aware that artificial sweeteners may raise your blood sugar levels.

Legumes

Legumes are beans, peas, and lentils, also known as pulses from the Latin word *puls*, which means bean porridge. The physical

---

Legumes: Low on the Glycemic Index

aduki (or adzuki) beans	lima beans
black beans	navy beans
black-eyed peas	pink beans
cowpeas	pinto beans
cranberry beans	red beans
garbanzo beans (chickpeas)	soybeans
great northern beans	split peas
kidney beans	white beans
lentils	

---

shape of the seeds distinguishes the type: dry beans are kidney-shaped or oval, peas are round, and lentils are flat disks.

Legumes slow down digestion and absorption of carbohydrates and minimize blood glucose elevation after you eat. When legumes replace meat and dairy foods in the meal plan, there is generally a reduction of total fat, saturated fatty acids, and cholesterol. This reduces the risk factors for **atherosclerosis**, a frequent complication for people with diabetes. (Mann 1985, Leeds 1981, Truswell 1994) Adding about three and a half ounces (dry weight) of legumes daily to the diabetic diet improves metabolic control and helps to control blood sugar over the long term.

Numerous clinical studies show that the soluble fibers in beans, peas, and lentils significantly reduce postprandial hyper-

Beans, Beans, the Musical Fruit . . .

Beans contain sugars called oligosaccharides that require a specific enzyme to break them down. Since the human digestive tract does not produce this enzyme, these compounds remain undigested and intestinal fermentation results in gas production and flatulence. Soaking, sprouting, and cooking the legumes can reduce this hard-to-digest sugar. Discarding the soaking and cooking water used to prepare the beans is the most effective way to remove these sugars. A product called Beano™ contains enzymes that break down the oligosaccharides. It is available in most health-food stores.

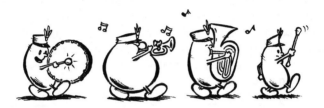

glycemia in individuals with type 1 and type 2 diabetes. Carefully controlled studies indicate that increased fiber intake, especially soluble fiber, reduces the rise in blood sugar after eating, improves insulin sensitivity, decreases LDL (**low-density lipoprotein**) cholesterol, and may have favorable effects on blood pressure and weight management.

Fiber in legumes affects how quickly food is absorbed, how fast the stomach empties into the intestines, intestinal motility and transit time, secretion rates and enzyme activity in the pancreas, short-chain fatty acid production in the colon, and secretion of intestinal and pancreative hormones.

NUTRITIONAL QUALITIES OF LEGUMES

All dry beans are remarkably similar in nutritional composition. A 100-gram portion is a half cup of dry beans, which provides about 350 calories. Beans contain 21 to 25 percent crude proteins, except for soybeans, with approximately 34 percent protein content. Soybean protein isolates used in protein powders,

---

Beans and the Little People

In the diabetic process, the little people need all the help they can get to make life easier. They love beans, peas, and lentils because these foods get broken down slowly, so the little people can work at a nice, even pace without the rush and confusion that happens when you eat a bowl of pasta, for example. The pasta, which is a refined carbohydrate, breaks down and gets absorbed within minutes, and the bloodstream workers get inundated with simple carbohydrates (sugar). They are also left with the daunting task of finding enough insulin and chromium to get each sugar molecule into a cell. The American Heart Association, the American Cancer Institute, and the American Diabetes Association all recommend a diet low in fat (no more than 30 percent of total calories), cholesterol (no more than 300 milligrams per day), and saturated fat (no more than 10 percent of calories). A meal plan based on whole plant foods (rich in legumes, whole grains, vegetables, and fruits) meets these recommendations.

---

now available in health-food stores, have essentially as much protein as meat. The total carbohydrate composition of dry beans ranges from 60 to 65 percent.

Vitamins and minerals. Dry beans are good sources of water-soluble vitamins, especially thiamine, riboflavin, niacin, folacin, vitamin E, and beta-carotene. Soybeans are also a substantial source of several minerals, including calcium, iron, copper, zinc, phosphorus, potassium, and magnesium.

Fat. The fat content of legumes is low, ranging from 1 to 15 percent. Soybeans, nuts, and seeds are exceptions: soybeans contain about 19 percent and nuts and seeds 46 percent fat. Because dry beans are plant foods, they are cholesterol free. The low lipid content of dry beans is especially important in light of recommendations suggesting that Americans lower their fat and cholesterol intakes to reduce risk of chronic disease. (Truswell 1994)

Fiber. Cooked dry beans contain a substantial amount of carbohydrate (3 to 7 percent) as fiber in the form of cellulose and hemicellulose. Fibers can be classified as either water soluble or water insoluble and are usually a mix of both. Beans are rich in soluble fiber, which significantly lowers blood cholesterol and blood glucose. The fiber in beans also helps the gastrointestinal tract function due to its bulking and binding properties and its hydration capacity (ability to combine with water). Legume fiber has more hydration capacity than whole-grain cereals.

Dry beans are an inexpensive, culinarily versatile, high-quality protein source, rich in complex carbohydrates, high in fiber, and an excellent source of vitamins and minerals. They stabilize blood sugar, lower cholesterol, and promote weight loss.

Fruits and Vegetables
Fruits and vegetables are our main sources of water-soluble vitamins and fiber, and legumes are our main source of protein. Produce should always be organic and fresh. Homegrown is ideal, but the second best option for high-quality produce is to buy local and seasonal so that the produce doesn't have to be shipped far. Foods that have been shipped long distances and stored lose some nutritional value due to oxidation from light and oxygen. Farmers' markets and the organic produce department at your local health-food store or co-op are good places to buy fresh, organic produce.

Whole fruits and vegetables contain several types of fiber, which help reduce cholesterol, clean out the intestines, and stimulate peristalsis, and these fresh foods provide the B vitamins we lose when we are under stress.

Beans, peas, and lentils are available canned or dried. Fresh legumes are ideal but not always available. The next best choice is dried, as they are inexpensive and have a lower glycemic index than canned beans. Dried beans are very important to the diabetic diet. Dried beans should be your main source of protein.

They can be cooked in soups, stews, and chilis or used cold in salads. Foods made from beans—such as the soybean products tempeh and tofu—can be used in smoothies, desserts, and salad dressings as egg, dairy, and meat alternatives.

Try to eat one to two pieces of fruit and six to eleven servings of fresh vegetables every day. Just one-half cup of vegetables counts as a serving. A large salad made with calcium-rich, dark-green leafy vegetables, such as spinach, a large red pepper, and a couple of carrots counts as five servings. Once you begin to eat fresh vegetables as a base part of each meal, you will find that it is easy to eat eleven servings of vegetables each day.

Fruits should always be eaten fresh and whole—not cooked or juiced, which softens and removes the fiber, consequently raising the glycemic index of these fruits. Without the fiber, the fruit sugars are absorbed too quickly and can cause a rise in blood sugar levels.

When choosing berries, remember that the deep colored berries, such as blackberries and boysenberries, have a very low glycemic index and are particularly good choices for blood sugar regulation.

There are hundreds of delicious fruits and vegetables to choose from in the grocery stores. Try a new one each week; this variety will keep you interested in preparing creative and healthy meals. The following lists categorize fruits and vegetables by their approximate glycemic indexes and indicate which ones may be eaten every day and which ones should be eaten only occasionally.

VEGETABLES TO EAT EVERY DAY

These vegetables have a glycemic index of 30 to 50 percent (except for soybeans, which are even lower). So load up on them.

black-eyed peas	(42)
chickpeas	(33)
kidney beans	(27)

lentils (29)

lima beans (32)

peas (22)

soybeans (10)

VEGETABLES TO MINIMIZE

These are a few vegetables that have just a little too much natural sugar content. They should be consumed only in small quantities with other foods.

beets (64)

carrots (71)

corn (popcorn, corn chips, canned corn) (59)

parsnip (97)

potatoes (98)

FRUITS TO EAT EVERY DAY

These fruits all have a glycemic index of 30 to 50 percent. Enjoy! Note that an asterisk indicates that the fruit is generally recognized as glycemically low.

apple (39)

applesauce (w/o added sugar or corn syrup) (34–42)

blackberries *

blueberries *

boysenberries *

cherries (22)

grapefruit (25)

grapes (43)

peach (28)

pear (33)

raspberries *

strawberries (32)

FRUITS TO MINIMIZE

banana (47–59)

dried fruits (60–69)

kiwi (46–58)

mango	(60)
pineapple	(59–73)
raisins	(60–69)
watermelon	(59–85)

Plant Fiber for Blood Sugar Regulation

Combining foods within the same meal mixes them in your stomach and changes the index for that entire meal. The goal is to stay between fifty and eighty on the index as much as possible. Eating a serving of fiber-rich beans and a glass of juice, for example, will not raise your blood sugar level as quickly as would a glass of juice on its own. This is also why sweets should be eaten with a meal and counted as part of the meal. Food with a longer digestive breakdown time, such as beans, will help the sugars be absorbed more slowly.

How Much Fiber Daily?

Most Americans do not eat enough fiber, as is evident from the frequency of such ailments as constipation, colon cancer, toxic bowels, and colon polyps. The average person gets only 8 to 10 measly grams of fiber in their diet per day. The RDA (**recommended dietary allowance**) is twenty-five to thirty-five grams per day, and people with diabetes should eat considerably more. Aim for sixty-five grams of fiber daily. Fiber is necessary for proper intestinal function. It works like a broom to clean out your intestines. Fiber also binds with excess cholesterol and helps to move it along and out of the body with waste products.

A Plant-Based Meal Plan for Blood Sugar Regulation

The plant-based meal plan consists of fruits, vegetables, legumes, grains, seeds, and nuts. Whole plant foods are as unrefined and unprocessed as possible. Fish and yogurt may be added to the diet in small quantities. Total vegetarianism is not necessary to reap the health benefits of a diet low in animal products; a plant-based diet has many of the same health benefits.

Fish oils are beneficial to people who are susceptible to heart disease—and since heart disease is America's number one killer, most of us are in that category. Fish oil lowers blood fat, prevents blood clots, reduces the likelihood of heart attack and stroke, and aids in reducing inflammation. Only recently have we begun to understand these important benefits of fish. Adding fish to a generally vegetarian meal plan stacks the cards in your favor.

Studies indicate that a vegetarian diet reduces mortality rates for several chronic degenerative diseases. (Butland 1988, Fraser 1988) These effects may be attributed to diet as well as lifestyle. Vegetarians tend to be nonsmokers who maintain a desirable weight, get regular exercise, and abstain from alcohol and recreational drugs.

Reducing animal products is healthy for many reasons. Mortality from **coronary artery** disease is lower in vegetarians than in nonvegetarians. (Butland 1988, Fraser 1988) Total serum **cholesterol** and LDL cholesterol levels are usually lower in vegetarians. (Kestin et al. 1989) Low-fat, low-cholesterol vegetarian diets may decrease levels of apoproteins A, B, and E; alter platelet composition and function; and decrease plasma viscosity.

Seventh-Day Adventist vegetarians have lower rates of mortality from colon cancer than the general population. (Phillips and Snowdon 1983) This may be attributed to their increased fiber intake; decreased intake of total fat, saturated fat, cholesterol, and caffeine; and increased intake of fruits and vegetables.

In short, the most effective diet for blood sugar control is rich in legumes, whole grains, vegetables, fruit, and fish and contains only minimal amounts of dairy products, red meat, and fowl.

Many factors affect glycemic response by delaying digestion and absorption of food:
- raw fruits and vegetables
- insoluble fiber, such as the fibrous coating on beans
- soluble fiber, like pectins, guar, phytates, and tannins
- smaller, more frequent meals

Taking control and accepting that your body has undergone change can be empowering and actually give you some very real health advantages in the long run. The healthy lifestyle changes necessary to control diabetes also reduce your risk of cancer, heart disease, and other autoimmune diseases. Use this disadvantage to face imbalances in your lifestyle and diet and improve your overall health. For example, create an exercise program that will reduce stress in your life, which will help protect you from other diseases. You may feel even better than you did before your diagnosis of diabetes.

A healthy meal plan for people with diabetes is basically a healthy diet for almost anyone. Your entire family, from athletes to overweight members, will benefit from this meal plan. When one person has diabetes, it is generally wise for others in the family, who may be predisposed to the disease, to follow the same diet.

Goals of the nutrition plan are these:

- Achieve and maintain blood glucose balance.
- Achieve optimal blood fat levels.
- Maintain a reasonable weight.
- Prevent complications.
- Provide for adequate physical growth in children and for growth of the fetus in pregnant women.

You can achieve these goals by doing the following:

- Eat close to the same times and the same quantities each day.
- Increase your intake of fiber.
- Increase complex carbohydrates.
- Increase your intake of whole foods (foods that are as unrefined and unprocessed as possible).
- Increase legumes (beans, peas, and lentils).
- Decrease simple carbohydrates.
- Decrease fats, especially saturated fats.
- Decrease cholesterol.

- Eliminate synthetic sweeteners.
- Reduce caffeine and alcohol.
- Decrease refined foods.
- Supplement with a multivitamin and mineral complex when needed.
- Get enough exercise.
- Reduce stress in your life.

The goal of managing diabetes is to keep blood sugar (glucose), blood cholesterol, triglyceride (lipid or fat), and blood pressure levels as close to normal as possible. Controlling diabetes can prevent diabetic complications. Current scientific literature substantiates the fact that a whole-foods, leguminous-fiber diet reduces health complications in people with diabetes. (Simpson et al. 1981)

The Basics of the Meal Plan

Let's take a closer look at the big four elements of the meal plan: increasing your intake of fiber, complex carbohydrates, whole plant foods, and legumes. As you'll see, the four interact. For example, when you eat beans, you're consuming fiber, complex carbohydrates, and a whole plant food (and, of course, a legume).

Increase fiber. Studies suggest that an increase in the intake of soluble fiber (to approximately 65 grams of dietary fiber daily) can lead to decreases in plasma glucose, glycosuria, insulin requirements, blood cholesterol levels, and serum lipoprotein risk factors for atherosclerosis. (Anderson and Ward 1979) Fiber is an important component due to its role in promoting gastrointestinal motility. High-fiber food sources include legumes, whole grains, bran products, nuts and seeds, vegetables, and fruit. Insoluble plant fiber is the portion of the plant food that is not broken down in the human digestive tract. (Anderson et al. 1987, Behall 1990) High-fiber foods are also the most effective way to stabilize blood sugar for people on oral diabetic agents (Kiehm et al. 1976) They enhance tissue sensitivity to insulin (as evidenced by an increase in insulin receptors on monocytes).

Increase complex carbohydrates. A large-scale study showed that high-carbohydrate and high-fiber diets containing sustained-release carbohydrates improved blood sugar control for diabetics. Many patients were able to reduce the insulin required daily, and some were even able to eliminate it. (Anderson 1979)

Increase plant foods. Whole plant foods are unrefined and unprocessed. By contrast, animal products do not contain fiber, are generally high in fat and cholesterol, can cause the artery walls to deteriorate, and often contain hormones and chemicals, which is why they are inappropriate protein sources. A combination of whole plant foods such as the popular high-carbohydrate, high-plant-fiber (HPF) diet devised by Dr. James Anderson has substantial validation in the scientific literature and is a good example of a whole-foods meal plan. (Simpson et al. 1981, Anderson 1979, Kay et al. 1981, and Vahouny and Kritchevsky 1982)

Increase legumes. A wide variety of legumes are available dried, which generally means they should be presoaked. Canned beans are precooked and just need reheating. Buy legumes without added sugar, salt, or preservatives. You can add dry beans to your diet gradually.

Because legumes are high in soluble and insoluble fiber, they are metabolized more slowly than refined or animal foods. This puts them lower on the glycemic index, which supports blood sugar control. Legumes are low in saturated fat, cholesterol, and sodium. They supply protein, complex carbohydrate, fiber, and essential vitamins and minerals. Beans help reduce the risk of many chronic diseases, including coronary heart disease, obesity, and cancer. Legumes are so good for you that they should be a major source of calories. (Anderson 1977, Anderson 1979,

Anderson 1992, Jenkins et al. 1994, Jenkins et al. 1980, Murray and Pizzorno 1991, Simpson et al. 1981, Vahouny and Kritchevsky 1982)

A high-carbohydrate, leguminous-fiber meal plan improves all aspects of diabetes control.

Dr. James Anderson of the Metabolic Research Group, Veterans' Affairs Medical Center in Diabetes Research and Clinical Practice

Edamame Recipe

This popular Japanese dish is a delicious way to prepare soybeans.

    1 frozen package of green soybeans
    1 teaspoon sea salt

Place soybeans in a bamboo steamer or a metal steamer basket. Steam for eight to ten minutes, until the beans are thawed and heated thoroughly. Just pull a bean out after eight minutes and taste. Shorter cooking time will keep them crisp, and longer cooking time will make them softer. When beans are cooked to desired consistency, remove from basket and place in a bowl. Sprinkle with sea salt and serve warm. To eat them, hold one end of the bean pod in your fingers and use your teeth to extract the tender beans inside. Do not eat the hull.

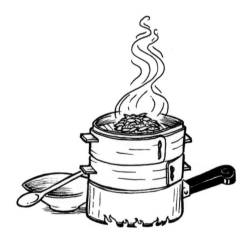

5

Understanding Fats

*F*ats, *lipids*, and *oils* are all terms used interchangeably for the same macronutrient, **fat**. Lipids are natural substances that will not dissolve in water. They include **triglycerides** and their breakdown products, the FAS (fatty acids), **phospholipids** (including lecithin), **lipoproteins**, and the **glycolipids**. Lipids are intimately related to the *fat-soluble vitamins* (A, D, E, and K), *coenzyme Q$_{10}$*, and the *steroid hormones*. The healthful foods that contain fat are fish, nuts, seeds, soybeans, and certain oils.

A diet high in unhealthful fats such as margarine, red meat, high-fat dairy products, and eggs increases the risk of coronary heart disease and obesity. Making small changes by choosing the right types of fats and keeping the overall quantity down, makes a big difference in the long run. For example, changing from whole milk to low-fat 2 percent milk reduces the fat content by almost 50 percent. Many people find that cutting out just one fatty food a day will result in weight loss within weeks. For example, if you have a cup of tea rather than your daily whole-milk latte, you will cut out 150 calories a day.

However, some types of fat are essential to our diet. Good fats help reduce cholesterol levels and provide the base materials our bodies need to make hormones and healthy tissues. For example, fish oils contain fatty acids that help keep cells whole, reduce inflammation, and build healthy tissue. Fish and fish oils are also recommended for the diabetic diet because hundreds of studies show they are high in omega-3 fatty acids, which lower triglyceride and cholesterol levels. There is evidence that a diet rich in omega-3 and omega-6 fatty acids may decrease insulin resistance and decrease the progression of microan-giopathy and cardiac ischemia. EFAS (**essential fatty acids**) support the function of the adrenal glands, aid in the metabolism of other fats, and prevent the buildup of **plaque** in the arteries. Individuals with glucose intolerance and **dyslipidemia** can greatly decrease their usually elevated triglyceride levels with omega-3 fatty acids.

Our country's leading health scientists now recommend increasing our intake of essential fatty acids while reducing our intake of **saturated fats**, and **trans fatty acids**. Evidence for the **atherogenic** potential of high-fat foods in those with diabetes has prompted the American Diabetes Association to recommend a fat intake of no more than 30 percent of total calories and a cholesterol intake of less than 300 milligrams per day. This is identical to the recommendations of the American Heart Association and the American Cancer Institute. For people who have diabetes and blood sugar disorders, 25 percent of total calories from fat is even better, but this is a lofty goal and we find that results with blood sugar regulation will be much the same up to 30 percent fat. In this program, we recommend a range of 25 to 30 percent fat. Keeping fat intake down takes some detective work and calculating.

Lipids, Fats, and Oils

Some fats are made by animals as a way of storing energy obtained from plants. All fats may contain the same number of calories per gram, but not all fats are created equal. Some fats are better than others. This chapter will help you distinguish between healthful fats and those that can be damaging to your health. Sometimes it is not the type of fats eaten but the amount that causes problems.

Lipids, fats, and *oils* are all words used interchangeably for the same nutrient. Technically, fats and oils (which are liquid fats) are part of a group of substances called **lipids**. In a general sense, lipids are organic (carbon-containing) substances that will not dissolve in water. Three major types of lipids are found in foods: triglycerides, phospholipids, and sterols. Other terms add to the confusion: saturated fats, polyunsaturated fats, omega-3 fats, monounsaturates, essential fatty acids, fish oil, cholesterol, EPA, DHA, GLA, and lecithin. These substances we are told, affect your LDL, HDL, and VLDL. All of these terms are freely used in conversation today, but few people really understand what they mean. To appreciate the important role lipids play in diabetes therapy, a little biochemistry is in order.

Fatty Acids

The basic building blocks of lipids are FAS (fatty acids), which are composed of carbon atoms arranged in a chain. At one end of the chain is a methyl group (CH_3) and at the other end is the carboxyl group (COOH).

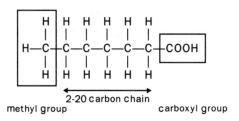

2-20 carbon chain
methyl group   carboxyl group

Composition of a fatty acid

Two smaller fatty acids can be joined together to produce a longer fatty acid if the methyl end of one is connected with the carboxyl group of the other. Fatty acids can be classified according to the degree of saturation, location of the first double bond, or length of the carbon chain.

Saturated and Unsaturated Fatty Acids

Each carbon atom in the carbon chain of a fatty acid has sites for two hydrogen atoms. When the carbon chain of a fatty acid has all the hydrogen atoms it can hold, it is said to be *saturated*. Saturated fats are very stable and do not go rancid easily. However, many saturated fats increase cholesterol production and blood cholesterol levels, so keep your intake to a minimum.

Butter is a natural fat that is high in saturated fatty acids. As you can see, the chain of a saturated fat is straight, making it easy for the molecules to remain stacked closely together. This makes the fat solid at room temperature.

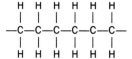

Saturated fatty-acid chain

When two hydrogen atoms are removed from two adjacent carbon atoms, these atoms use the available sites to add another bond between them, making it a *double bond*. A fatty acid with one double bond is said to be a MUFA (**monounsaturated fatty acid**) because *mono* means one.

The double bond also causes a kink in the chain. This makes it difficult to stack the chains, like trying to stack folded chairs on top of one chair that is partly open. They fall around each other, and this is what makes the fat a liquid. As the percentage of MUFAs increases, a fat becomes more fluid.

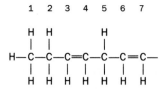

Monounsaturated fatty acid

In longer carbon chains, more than one double bond may be formed. These fatty acids are called PUFAs (**polyunsaturated fatty acids**) because *poly* means many. The PUFA shown here has two double bonds. (Notice the double line between the third and fourth carbon atoms from the left.)

```
        1   2   3   4   5   6   7

        H   H           H
        |   |           |
    H—C—C—C═C—C—C═C—
        |   |   |   |   |   |   |
        H   H   H   H   H   H   H
```

Polyunsaturated fatty acid

The double bonds in PUFAs are very vulnerable to attack from oxygen in the air. The addition of oxygen (oxidation) causes changes in flavor and odor that are commonly called **rancidity**. In large doses, rancid oils can be toxic. To prevent oxidation, some PUFAs have hydrogen added to the double-bonded carbons, breaking the additional bond and making the fatty acid more stable. This is called **hydrogenation**.

Hydrogenated oils are solid at room temperature. The greater the degree of saturation, the more solid a fat becomes; the lower the saturation, the more liquid it becomes. Tub margarines have less saturation than those that come in sticks.

$$
\begin{array}{ccccc}
\overset{\displaystyle \mid \;\; \mid}{\underset{\displaystyle \mid \;\; \mid}{-C=C-}} & + & H_2 & = &
\overset{\displaystyle H \;\; H}{\overset{\displaystyle \mid \;\; \mid}{\underset{\displaystyle \mid \;\; \mid}{\underset{\displaystyle H \;\; H}{-C-C-}}}} \\
\text{H \;\; H} & & & &
\end{array}
$$

unsaturated + hydrogen = hydrogenated fatty acid

Hydrogenation

When fatty acids are hydrogenated, they increase the saturation of fats. A high intake of saturated fats is a risk factor for many diseases. Also, trans isomers of unsaturated fats appear. These trans fatty acids do not function like normal FAs, and they are linked with an increase in heart disease.

Omega Number of Fatty Acids

The location of the *first* double bond is another way of classifying fatty acids. This location is found by counting from the methyl end of the molecule. For example, look at the earlier figure of the polyunsaturated fatty acid. The first double bond is found on the third carbon atom, so its omega number (ω) is 3. Oils rich in **omega-3 fatty acids** are often in the news these days.

Three important omega-3 fatty acids are EPA **(eicosapentaenoic acid)**, DHA **(docosahexaenoic acid)**, and LNA **(linolenic acid)**. Linolenic acid is one of the two essential fatty acids. They're called essential because the body cannot manufacture them; they must be obtained from the diet. The body can manufacture both EPA and DHA from linolenic acid, but often it does not manufacture enough. By adding supplemental EPA and DHA through fish oil, you can enjoy the benefits of these fatty acids. The omega-3 fatty acids lower blood triglyceride levels, decrease platelet stickiness, and keep the arteries clean from fatty deposits. How this is done is not well understood. Unlike chicken (which should be eaten with the skin removed), fish should be eaten with the skin on to get the most of these fats.

The **omega-6 fatty acids** also have unique properties. They include LA **(linoleic acid)**, the other essential amino acid; AA **(arachidonic acid)**, which is manufactured from linoleic acid; and GLA **(gamma linolenic acid)**. GLA is manufactured as a result of the first step toward the production of hormone-like substances called *prostaglandins*, but not everyone manufactures enough GLA. Good sources of GLA supplements are evening primrose oil and borage seed oil.

Young children need more EFAs than adults and males need more than females. Older infants who are fed low-fat cow's milk can develop an EFA deficiency.

Chain Length of Fatty Acids

Fatty acids are also described by the length of their carbon chain. Formic acid (released in bee stings and ant bites) has only one carbon atom. Acetic acid (vinegar) has two carbon atoms. Since these FAs are so short, they are soluble in water, which makes them act more like water-soluble acids. The fatty acids found in food range from four carbons (butyric acid) to twenty-four (found in fish oils).

Within this range, fatty acids are described as having short, medium, or long chains.

- Short-chain FAs contain two to six carbon atoms. They are found in butter and milk.

- Medium-chain FAS contain eight to twelve carbon atoms. They are very easy to absorb and are available as medium-chain triglycerides (MCTS) at pharmacies. Coconut is very rich in MCTS.
- Long-chain FAS contain sixteen or more carbon atoms.

carbon numbers

| 1 | 2 | 3 | 4 | 5 | 6 | 7 | 8 | 9 | 10 | 11 | 12 | 13 | 14 | 15 | 16 | 17 | 18 |

$$\begin{array}{c} \text{H} \mid \text{H} \quad \text{H} \quad \text{H} \quad \text{H} \quad \text{H} \quad \text{H} \quad \text{H} \quad \text{H} \quad \text{H} \quad \text{H} \quad \text{H} \quad \text{H} \quad \text{H} \quad \text{H} \quad \text{H} \quad \text{H} \\ \text{H—C}\mid\text{C—C=C—C—C=C—C—C=C—C—C—C—C—C—C—C}\mid\text{COOH} \\ \text{H} \mid \text{H} \qquad \text{H} \qquad \text{H} \qquad \text{H} \quad \text{H} \quad \text{H} \quad \text{H} \quad \text{H} \quad \text{H} \end{array}$$

← carbon chain →

methyl group   carboxyl group

Linolenic acid

Let's see how to classify a molecule of linolenic acid. We know it is a fatty acid because it follows the formula: a methyl group at one end, a carboxyl group at the other, and two to twenty-four carbons in between. It has three double bonds, which makes it a polyunsaturated fatty acid. It has eighteen carbon atoms, so it is a long-chain FA, with double bonds at carbon numbers 3, 6, and 9. This makes its omega number 3. A shorthand description of this molecule is 18: 3 ω 3. This represents eighteen carbon molecules and three double bonds, with the first double bond (counting from the methyl group) at carbon number 3.

Linolenic acid has a cis configuration. *Cis* and *trans* are descriptions of the arrangement of hydrogen atoms around the double bonds. In nature, both of the hydrogen atoms on the double-bonded carbons are on the same side of the molecule. The shape of a molecule determines its function. If you alter the shape, you alter the function. Molecules that are trans versions do not have the same effect in the body as the natural cis version. This has been demonstrated with trans fatty acids found in margarines and spreads; they elevate cholesterol at least as much as saturated fats.

Types of Lipids

Up to now we have considered only fatty acids. How are they related to the everyday fats and oils we are familiar with? In general, they combine to form lipids (fats) in food.

Triglycerides

Most of the lipids in foods are triglycerides. Triglycerides are composed of four molecules: the glycerol molecule, which acts as a three-"rod" hanger, and the three (tri) fatty acids that hang from each rod. The properties and abilities of each triglyceride depend on the characteristics of its component fatty acids.

$$
\begin{array}{l}
\text{H} \\
|\\
\text{H—C—OH} \\
|\\
\text{OH—C—H} \quad + \quad 3(\text{R—COOH}) \\
|\\
\text{H—C—OH} \\
|\\
\text{H}
\end{array}
\quad = \quad
\begin{array}{l}
\text{H} \\
|\\
\text{H—C—OOC—R1} \\
|\\
\text{R2—COO—C—C} \\
|\\
\text{H—C—OOC—R3} \\
|\\
\text{H}
\end{array}
$$

glycerol   +   3 fatty acids   =   triglyceride

Formation of a triglyceride

For example, the properties of an oil are related to the types of triglycerides found in that oil. In turn, the properties of triglycerides are determined by the fatty acids that form it, and the properties of the fatty acids are determined by their structure. The longer and more unsaturated the fatty acids, the more liquid or soft the fat is at room temperature. The order of the fatty acids on the glycerol molecule also affects the digestibility and absorbability of the triglyceride. Because there are so many different fatty acids in natural foods, there are many types of triglycerides in a fat or oil.

Monoglycerides (with one fatty acid hanging on the glycerol) and *diglycerides* (with two fatty-acid molecules) are also found in foods. They too are produced during the digestion of triglycerides.

Sterols

Another familiar group of lipids is the **sterols**. The most infamous sterol is cholesterol, which is found only in animal foods and is manufactured in the liver. Not all bad, cholesterol is the precursor for steroids, including bile acids and the sex hormones. In the liver it can be converted to the precursor of vitamin D, it waterproofs the skin, and it is necessary for proper brain development in infants. *Beta sitosterol*, found in rice bran, competes with cholesterol for absorption, so it reduces blood cholesterol levels.

Compound Lipids

The final group of lipids has the following members:

- *Phospholipids* are compounds of fatty acids, phosphoric acid, and a nitrogen-containing base. Lecithin is one of the most common phospholipids.
- *Glycolipids* are compounds of fatty acids, carbohydrate, and a nitrogen-containing base. Glycolipids are part of nerve tissue and certain cell membranes.
- *Sulpholipids* are lipids that contain sulfur.
- *Lipoproteins* are lipids combined with protein. Well-known lipoproteins include **chylomicrons**, the droplets in which lipids are packaged to travel in the lymph system to the bloodstream; VLDLS **(very low-density lipoproteins)**, the transport packages for triglycerides in the blood; LDLs (low-density lipoproteins), which carry cholesterol to the tissues and are commonly referred to as "bad" cholesterol; and HDLS **(high-density lipoproteins)**, the "good" cholesterol that removes cholesterol from the tissues and brings it back to the liver.
- *Lipopolysaccharides* are lipids that contain polysaccharides.

Lipid Storage

Humans have two types of body fat: brown and white. Most fat is white. It is made of **adipose cells** that accumulate beneath the skin, around internal organs, and inside muscle tissue. These fat cells store fat as liquid triglycerides.

Brown adipose tissue occurs in much smaller amounts. It decreases with age and is involved in *thermogenesis*, the creation of heat. Brown fat produces energy to warm the body in response to cold.

Functions of Lipids

Although we have a tendency to consider lipids bad, they are necessary for human life. Their functions include the following:

- Fats are the most concentrated form of energy. They provide nine calories for every gram burned, which is more than twice as much energy per gram as carbohydrates or proteins.
- Adipose (fat) tissue holds organs in place, and the subcutaneous (below the skin) layer of fat provides insulation from the cold and maintains body temperature.
- Fat spares the B vitamin thiamine, which is needed so you can use carbohydrate for energy.
- Fat spares protein. When fat is present, the body does not have to burn protein for fuel.
- Fat helps in the absorption and transport of the fat-soluble vitamins A, D, E, and K.
- Lipids slow the rate at which foods leave the stomach. This means that the carbohydrate also present is not released all at once, which would cause insulin and blood sugar levels to rise. Fats decrease the appetite, giving the feeling of satiety.
- Fat makes foods more palatable.
- Lipids provide the building blocks of sterols, prostaglandins, thromboxanes, prostacyclins, and cell membranes.

Metabolism of Lipids

Fat molecules are too large to be absorbed directly and must be broken down into smaller units. The enzymes responsible for lipid digestion are called *lipases* (*lipo* = fat, *ase* = enzyme). Gastric lipase (*gastric* = stomach) partially emulsifies and digests the short- and medium-chain fatty acids, and many are absorbed before they have a chance to reach the small intestine.

When fats are detected in the duodenum, *bile* made in the liver is secreted into the small intestine. Bile is an emulsifying agent. It breaks fat into small lipid droplets in the same way shampoo emulsifies the oils in your hair. This makes lipids, mainly long-chain fatty acids, more accessible to the lipases secreted by the pancreas. They are digested to produce monoglycerides, diglycerides, and free fatty acids, which are absorbed into the intestinal wall and then reassembled on the other side into triglycerides.

These triglycerides are packaged into chylomicrons for transport by the lymphatic system, bypassing the portal vein that takes the water-soluble compounds to the liver. Lymph vessels bring them to the left shoulder, where they are discharged into the bloodstream. Chylomicrons are large enough to make plasma look "milky" after a fat-rich meal.

Medium-chain triglycerides (MCTs) have a chain eight to ten carbons in length. MCTs need very little lipase and no bile to be digested. Unlike the long chains, they do not need to be reassembled into triglycerides after absorption. They easily dissolve into the blood and are carried via the portal vein to the liver. Because they bypass the slow-moving lymph system, MCTs are absorbed as fast as glucose. They are an excellent source of energy for people who have damage to their intestinal villi due to malnutrition, radiation, or chemotherapy or who lack sufficient pancreatic enzymes or bile acids. Pure MCT in oil form can be purchased in pharmacies without a prescription but should only be added to the diet with the guidance of a nutritional expert such as a naturopathic physician who will assess your individual need for, and the appropriate dose of, MCT supplementation. It is not very palatable and must be mixed with food—for example, soy milk blended with banana.

A Guide to Fats and Oils

Be aware of the sources of fat in your meal plan. There is fat in seeds, nuts, avocados, olives, and salad dressings, so eat these foods in moderation. Be sure you are getting healthful oils (essential fatty acids) that your body does not manufacture on its own. Fish and flaxseed oil are both good sources of EFAS. All oils should be unrefined and expeller-pressed, not chemically extracted. Buy organic oils whenever possible. Oils often contain unhealthy quantities of pesticides and herbicides. Soybean and canola oil are two products that have unusually high levels of residues. To avoid these toxic chemicals buy only certified organic products. Spectrum Naturals, Inc. is one high-quality, widely distributed, culinary oil company that sells organic oils.

Fat Sources to Include in Your Daily Meal Plan

The following fats are so good for you that you should make a point of eating them every day.

- *Borage seed oil* is an excellent source of EFAS with gamma linolenic acid. Borage oil contains twice as much GLA as evening primrose oil.
- *Canola oil* contains omega-3, -6, and -9 fatty acids and is rich in vitamins K and E.
- *Evening primrose oil* is sold as a supplement in liquid and capsule forms. It is a high-quality source of EFAS, but it is fairly expensive. It contains GLA (though not nearly as much as borage oil).
- *Extra-virgin olive oil* is the first press from the olives and does not require chemicals in the extraction process. Use it as a base for salad dressings.

Healthful Sources of Fat

Nuts

almonds and almond milk	filberts
beechnuts	hazelnuts
Brazil nuts	peanuts
cashews	pecans
chestnuts	walnuts

Seeds

flaxseeds	sesame seeds
pumpkin seeds	sunflower seeds

Oils

extra-virgin olive oil	safflower oil
flaxseed oil	

Soy Products

soy cheese	soy nuts
soy flour	tofu
soy milk	

- *Fish oils* are rich in omega-3 fatty acids. Eat fish every day. Include grilled salmon, tuna fish sandwiches, baked trout, and stir-fry with fish fillets.
- *Flaxseed oil* is high in omega-3 fatty acids. One tablespoon each day should be enough if fish and/or nuts are also a part of your daily meal plan. If flaxseed oil is your only daily EFA source, take one tablespoon twice a day. Buy only flax oil that is high quality, certified organic, unrefined fresh-pressed, and made by a reputable company such as Omega Nutrition or Arrowhead Mills.
- *Safflower oil* is rich in polyunsaturated fatty acids and linoleic acid, but it is low in omega-3 FAS. This makes it somewhat less healthful than flax oil.

- *Sesame oil* has traditionally been used in Asian and Middle Eastern cooking. It has such a distinctive flavor that it is generally used in small amounts as a flavoring. Sesame oil is rich in MUFAS and PUFAS.
- *Sunflower oil* is a rich source of PUFAS and vitamin E.
- *Other vegetable oils*, such as peanut, hazelnut, and almond, can be healthful if they are not too heavily processed.

Fats You Can Eat Occasionally

Some fats can be indulged in occasionally. Don't eat the items on this list too often, and look for the least processed versions of them.

- *Butter* is made from dairy milk and can be used in small amounts if enough EFAS are present in your diet. Because butter is solid, light and oxygen don't make it deteriorate and it can be used for cooking.
- *Cheese* is formed when rennin (the enzymes from a cow's stomach) is used to curdle or harden milk products. Cheese is generally made from dairy milk, so it contains any hormones the cow has been injected with and pesticides it has been exposed to. Most cheeses are high in fat, saturated fat, and cholesterol. Look for strong-tasting hard cheeses, such as Parmesan and hot-pepper flavored, and use them only as a condiment, not as a main part of a meal. You can also find cheese products made without rennin in health-food stores.
- *Eggs* contain about five grams of fat and 213 to 250 milligrams of cholesterol, and the yolks are 79 percent total fat. Use just the egg whites most of the time; use yolks occasionally as part of a meal.
- *Ghee* is clarified butter whose protein and impurities have been removed. The oil left behind is 100 percent animal fat. Ghee does not smoke when cooked or develop toxic compounds if overheated. It is a healthier choice than butter but must be used in moderation. Ghee has been used in India for thousands of years.

- *Red meat* should be used sparingly. Get most of your protein from fish and beans. If you crave red meat, choose lean cuts and have an ounce or two as a condiment rather than as your main protein source.
- *Shrimp* and *shellfish* contain cholesterol and lipids. They are also the filters of the sea, so they often have concentrations of the pollutants and heavy metals now in our oceans. You can eat small quantities of clams, mussels, oysters, and scallops occasionally, but fish is a safer source of EFAS.

Fat and Cholesterol Sources to Avoid

The items on this list have almost no redeeming qualities. Try to eliminate them entirely from your meal plan.

- *Bacon* is high in saturated fat and cholesterol. When charred until crisp, it also contains the carcinogens created when fats are burned.
- *Breads* made from refined flours (not just white bread) have had much of their fiber removed. Refined breads are metabolized so quickly that the carbohydrates become sugars within minutes, which elevates blood sugar levels.
- *Corn oil* is not recommended as a source of fatty acids. Corn has such low oil content that high temperatures and toxic solvents are needed to extract the oil efficiently.
- *Fried foods* are usually fried in unsaturated oil. But when unsaturated oil is heated and exposed to air and light, it undergoes rapid changes and produces many toxic substances, such as trans fatty acids.
- *Gravies* and *sauces* are generally made from animal fat in the form of melted lard, with white flour as a thickener. They are best avoided, especially in restaurants or social situations where you do not know their exact ingredients.
- *Hydrogenated oils* and *shortenings* contain altered molecules and fatty-acid fragments that may be toxic. Hydrogenated fats have been implicated in heart disease and should be avoided. (See "Hydrogenation and the Evils of Margarine" later in this chapter.)

- *Ice cream* usually contains sugar, cream, and preservatives. Avoid store-bought ice cream and consider making your own with the herb stevia as the sweetener, nonfat milk, and low-glycemic fruits like blueberries.
- *Lard* is animal fat from meats. Bacon fat, fatty cuts of red meat, organ meats, salami, and gravies are all laden with lard. It contains concentrated cholesterol and saturated fats and should be avoided.
- *Margarine* is hydrogenated vegetable oil. Hydrogen has been added to solidify the oil, which extends its shelf life. Hydrogenation turns the fat into trans fatty acids, which contribute to heart disease, cancer, and high cholesterol levels. Butter is a healthier choice than margarine, but ghee is even better.
- *Organ meats* like kidney and liver are filtering organs, so they contain a high concentration of toxic waste materials. They are also usually high in fat and cholesterol.
- *Palm* and *coconut oils* are extracted with poisonous solvents such as hexane, and most of their vital nutrients are destroyed in the processing. The raw forms of these oils are rich in beta-carotene, vitamin E, and the omega fatty acids, but the raw forms are not currently available in the United States. Because of their fatty-acid composition (which makes them semisolid at room temperature without needing hydrogenation) and their resistance to oxidation, they are often used in baked goods.

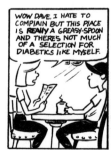
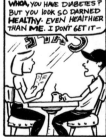
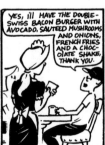
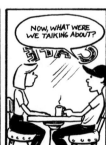

- *Pastries* from the store are loaded with butterfat and sugar and often with hydrogenated oils. You can make low-fat, whole-grain cookies and cakes and use an herbal sweeter like stevia.

- *Processed foods* in general should be avoided. The refining process often oxidizes fats and depletes foods of their fiber, vitamins, and minerals.

- *Red meats* like beef, lamb, and pork are high in fat and often contain synthetic hormones. They also have a lot of cholesterol and no fiber. Fatty cuts of red meat are basically lard deposits, filled with saturated fatty acids, cholesterol, and extra fat calories. Substitute fish and legumes as protein sources.

- *Salad dressings* are America's number one source of fat. Most dressings are made from hydrogenated oils. Always read the label before you buy, and choose dressings made from extra-virgin olive oil. Or make your own from flaxseed oil.

- *Salami* and *other cured meats* (such as sausage, hot dogs, and lunch meats) contain a lot of fat, sodium, and cancer-causing chemicals like nitrates. Try the soy-based, chemical-free hot dogs and lunch meats that are now available in many health-food stores.

- *Saturated fats* are hard at room temperature. They are prevalent in meats, butter, margarine, cheese, sour cream, and coconut oil, among other food products. Saturated fats can be converted to cholesterol by the liver.

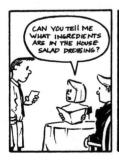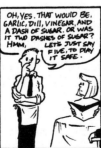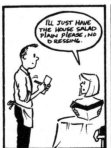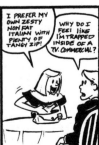

- *Shortenings* include lard products, butter, and hydrogenated vegetable oils such as Crisco. They carry the same risk factors as margarine and should be avoided.
- *Soy oil* is exposed to high temperatures and toxic solvents in the extraction process. Whole soy foods are superior to oil.
- *Walnut oil* products are often heavily processed and refined and are best avoided. Only certain varieties of walnuts have omega-3 and omega-6 fatty acids.
- *Whole milk* has dramatically more fat than skim milk. The chart compares the fat and calorie contents of an eight-ounce glass of whole and skim milk.

Fat and Calorie Content of Milk

	Whole Milk	2% Milk	Skim Milk
Calories	150	120	85
Protein (grams)	8	8.1	8.4
Carbohydrates (grams)	11.3	11.7	11.8
Fiber	0	0	0
Total fat (grams)	8.2	4.7	0.4
Saturated fat (grams)	5.0	2.9	0.3
Unsaturated fat (grams)	2.7	1.5	0.1
Cholesterol (milligrams)	33	18	0.4

Oil Dos and Don'ts

Once oils have been extracted, they will not store well. They must be kept refrigerated and away from light and oxygen to preserve them as long as possible. Store oils in the refrigerator in airtight, light-excluding containers. (Heat, light, or air will oxidize oils.) When oils are **oxidized**, their properties are changed. They no longer have a healthful effect and can even be very harmful.

Buy only fresh oils because rancid oils are altered and contain **free radicals**, which can contribute to cancer and heart disease. Rancid oils smell like fish or like the children's clay Play-

Doh. When they begin to get rancid, throw them out. One trick for keeping air away from oils is to add clean marbles to the container as the oil is used. The marbles replace the space that air would fill by keeping the level of oil up to the lid. When the oil is used up, the jar will be full of marbles. Put all the marbles in a mesh bag and run them through the dishwasher for future use.

Do not purchase oil in metal containers because contaminants will be leached from the metal and solder. Buy organic oils only. Omega Nutrition, Arrowhead Mills, and Spectrum Naturals, Inc. have third party–certified organic oil in light-excluding containers. Avoid all products that contain lard, hydrogenated oils, or margarine.

Even though fats have that smooth texture and great flavor that we are all accustomed to in our Western diets, they are also notorious for contributing to many of the diseases we now face. Also, fat tends to stick around—on hips, thighs, and waists, in arteries, and all the places we least want it. We do, however, need a certain amount of fat for our bodies to continue their important functions. These fats are best derived from natural, organic sources. Remember that any oil that is solid at room temperature is probably saturated and possibly hydrogenated, so it should be avoided.

The best bottled oils to have in your kitchen are flaxseed oil (for using raw) and olive oil for cooking.

Hydrogenation and the Evils of Margarine

One study reported in the *American Journal of Clinical Nutrition* illustrates the deleterious effects of margarine and hydrogenated fats in our diets. The study monitored two villages in India. The northern population was consuming meat and butter as their main fat source. They had high cholesterol levels, as would be expected. The southern group was vegetarian; they consumed hydrogenated fats such as margarine but no meats or dairy products. Yet the vegetarian group had fifteen times as much heart disease as their northern neighbors. The major dietary difference, noted by the doctor who performed the study, was that the southerners gave up the traditional natural use of ghee (clarified butter) for margarine and refined polyunsaturated vegetable oils.

Food scientists point out that a molecule of hydrogenated fat looks very much like a molecule of plastic. One of the reasons biochemists study the molecular shapes of substances is because their shapes define their functions. These plasticlike molecules are not recognized as natural by your body. If an altered fat molecule takes the place of an essential fat in your membrane structure, the result is that your membrane has a faulty structure and can no longer function properly. Hydrogenation of oils has been one of the most profound and health-damaging experiments in our food supply in the twentieth century. We can choose not to be a part of this experiment by avoiding hydrogenated foods.

Better Butter Recipe

½ cup butter

½ cup extra-virgin olive oil

Combine the butter and oil in a food processor or blender. Mix thoroughly and pour into a container with a lid. Store in the refrigerator and use it just as you would use butter. Better butter has half the saturated fat and half the cholesterol of full dairy butter. But remember, it is still 100 percent fat, so use it sparingly.

6

Proteins and the

Glycemic Index

*A*fter you eat protein foods and they break down into **amino acids**, they can float around in your bloodstream building and repairing hormones and tissues for up to seventy-two hours.

Protein foods affect blood sugar in many ways. Carbohydrates induce insulin output, and insulin promotes fat storage. Proteins, on the other hand, promote the mobilization and utilization of stored energy that burns fat.

People with type 1 diabetes are in a catabolic state without insulin replacement. Insulin's anticatabolic effect has been investigated in studies, which found increases in both protein breakdown and protein synthesis during insulin deprivation. Because there is a greater increase in protein breakdown than in protein synthesis, protein deprivation can result. Studies show that insulin replacement inhibits protein breakdown and synthesis in certain tissues. It appears that insulin exerts its overall anti-catabolic effect in insulin-dependent diabetes mainly by inhibiting the breakdown of muscle protein.

Protein in the form of high-fiber, nutrient-dense, low-glycemic legumes should be eaten every day. Many canned beans and dried peas range from 40 to 49 percent on the glycemic index, while chickpeas, black-eyed peas, and haricot beans range from 30 to 39 percent. Kidney beans and lentils are even better choices for blood sugar regulation, as they are low on the glycemic index and range from 20 to 29 percent. Soybeans, which have cancer-fighting chemicals and plant estrogens which help relieve menopausal symptoms, are very low on the glycemic index, as are peanuts at 10 to 19 percent.

Shapes of Protein Molecules

There are twenty-two different amino acids in the human body. Each amino acid is joined to another by means of a *peptide bond* to form *peptide* or *polypeptide chains*. Chemically, each amino acid is composed of an amino group (*amine* = contains nitrogen), a carboxyl group (*oxyl* = contains oxygen), a hydrogen atom, and the rest of the molecule, R, which differentiates it from other types. The R group can range from twenty-three to several hundred thousand amino groups.

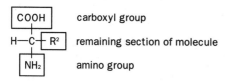

COOH — carboxyl group

H—C—R² — remaining section of molecule

NH₂ — amino group

Amino acid

The twenty-two amino acids identified in the body form a sort of alphabet. Each amino acid "letter" can be used to make up an unlimited number of protein words.

What your body does with the protein is determined by the protein's shape. Chains of polypeptides are twisted together to form a coil that resembles a Slinky toy. The hydrogen atoms in the Slinky form an effective but weak bond between turns of the coil. As long as the hydrogen bonds are intact, the protein holds its coil shape. These coils are then arranged into a specific shape that determines what the body uses it for.

Simple but long arrangements called *fibrous proteins* are used to make structural parts of tissue. These include the collagen in connective tissue, the keratin in hair and nails, and the myosin in muscles. Fibrous proteins do not dissolve in water and are very strong structurally.

If the chain is twisted after it forms a Slinky, it folds into itself, making a kind of knot. In a peptide coil, this knot is held in place by the sulfur-to-sulfur bonds found in some of the amino acids. Slinky knots are called *globular proteins*. They form enzymes and are present in the extracellular fluid of plants and animals. They dissolve easily in water. Globular proteins are found in egg whites, the casein of milk, the hemoglobin of red blood cells, and the albumins and globulins of blood plasma.

When a protein enters the digestive tract, it cannot be absorbed until it has been broken down into its amino acid components. This is done by *hydrolysis*, the breakage of peptide bonds by the addition of a molecule of water. This produces smaller proteins: individual amino acids, dipeptides (two amino acid proteins), and tripeptides (three amino acid proteins), which are easily absorbed by the digestive tract. The reverse is also true: a peptide bond is formed when a molecule of water is removed from two adjacent amino acids.

Formation of a peptide bond (one dipeptide) when water is removed

Hydrolysis (breakage of a peptide bond when water is added, forming two peptides)

This peptide bond can easily be attacked by the digestive enzymes of bacteria. Such bacterial growth, and formation of potentially toxic proteins as a by-product, causes food spoilage. This is why protein foods—such as milk, eggs, meat, poultry, and fish—must be refrigerated.

Types of Amino Acids

The body can manufacture most of the amino acids it needs from carbohydrate, fat, and other amino acids. These *nonessential amino acids* are essential for life; they are nonessential only in the sense that they do not have to be obtained from the diet.

Eleven other amino acids cannot be manufactured in amounts needed to support growth and maintenance. These *essential amino acids* must be obtained from the diet. Without them, protein cannot be made and body tissues cannot be maintained.

Protein and the Little People

The amino acids that are necessary for building skin, hair, hormones, enzymes, and many of your body's chemicals and tissues come from protein foods. The little people who make all of these tissues and chemicals need high-quality building blocks to make high-quality cells, hormones, and so on. Protein foods are meat, dairy products, eggs, fish, and beans. But because red meat, dairy, and eggs also have unhealthful qualities, they are best used only in small quantities.

Fish is an excellent source of protein; it provides all of the essential amino acids and the much-needed essential fatty acids. The little people like their protein in the form of legumes, which are high in fiber and break down slowly. This gives them a nice, evenly paced workday—no rushing around trying to deal with lots of fats and sugars in the bloodstream. Make it easy on your little people and provide them with at least one serving of beans each and every day.

Functions of Amino Acids

Besides forming the building blocks of protein, each amino acid has other specific functions in the body. *Tryptophan* is a *precursor* of (used to make) both the B vitamin niacin and serotonin, a neurotransmitter in the brain. *Methionine* provides sulfur groups for protein manufacture and detoxification of toxins by the liver. *Phenylalanine* is a precursor of the amino acid *tyrosine*, which is used to make hair and skin pigment. *Histadine* is used to make histamine, a chemical that dilates blood vessels, and glycine, which combines with toxic chemicals and makes them harmless. *Glutamic acid* is a precursor of *gamma-aminobutyric acid* (GABA), a neurotransmitter.

Complete and Incomplete Protein

The concept of "complete" and "incomplete" protein is one of the most confusing notions in nutrition. It was developed in an age when animal protein was considered the gold standard of protein quality. Today the ideas of complete and incomplete protein have taken on an entirely new meaning.

The so-called *complete proteins* contain all nine of the essential amino acids in sufficient quantities to allow growth in a young animal. Not surprisingly, ovalbumin (the main protein in egg) and casein (the main protein in milk) are complete proteins. The protein found in animal flesh is also complete. In the unlikely event that you had to depend on only a single food to survive, it would have to be a complete protein source. This condition, however, rarely occurs except in infancy.

The amino acids obtained from the diet are combined in the body with amino acids recycled from internal tissue breakdown. It is from this amino acid pool that the tissues draw their protein for new cells. The notion of protein combining—the belief that complementary proteins must be eaten at the same meal or a protein deficiency will ensue—has been thoroughly disproved.

Complete proteins also come packaged with "complete fats." Since saturated fat is an absolute necessity for infant brain development and growth, complete protein foods are likely to be excellent sources of unneeded, artery-clogging saturated fats.

Incomplete proteins lack these saturated fats. Like the complete proteins, they contain all nine of the essential amino acids. The only difference is that the amounts of these amino acids differ from food to food, in much the same way that vitamin and mineral levels vary.

Incomplete protein sources are superior to complete protein sources. Plant proteins are usually low in total fat and saturated fat and free of cholesterol. The high-fat sources of incomplete protein, such as nuts and seeds, contain heart-healthy fats. They are also excellent sources of fiber, minerals, vitamins, and phytochemicals.

Nitrogen Balance

True protein deficiencies are very rare and do not occur in healthy, well-nourished individuals. *Protein-calorie malnutrition* is due to lack of enough food to maintain health. This can result from much higher than normal protein needs or an inability to absorb the protein that is eaten.

Nitrogen balance is a term you are likely to hear your physician or nutritionist use. Since protein is the only nitrogen-containing macronutrient, the amount of nitrogen in the body is an accurate method of determining protein content of the body. When the amount of protein in the diet is known and the amount of protein being excreted is known, then the amount of protein left in the body can be measured.

When nitrogen intake and nitrogen output are equal, a person is said to be in nitrogen balance or equilibrium. This is the usual state for healthy adults.

A person who has more nitrogen coming in than going out is in *positive nitrogen balance*. This means that the buildup of tissue is greater than the breakdown of tissue. This occurs in pregnant and lactating mothers, growing infants, children, and adolescents, and adults who are recovering from an illness that resulted in a protein loss.

A *negative nitrogen balance* means the opposite is happening. There is more nitrogen leaving than coming in; the rate of tissue breakdown is greater than the rate of tissue synthesis. This occurs when 1) the body is not taking in enough protein, 2) protein is being burned for energy because not enough fat and carbohydrates are present for fuel, or 3) the protein needs of the body are greatly increased, as in some serious illnesses.

Protein in Your Meal Plan

How should you integrate this important macronutrient into your meal plan? The following lists provide some guidelines.

Protein Foods to Eat Daily

Legumes should comprise the bulk of your daily protein requirement.

- legumes (beans, peas, lentils)
- fish (fresh, canned, or frozen) such as salmon, halibut, snapper, orange roughy
- shellfish (shrimp, lobster, scampi, scallops, oysters, clams)
- yogurt (plain, low-fat)
- nuts and seeds
- soy products (tofu, soy milk, soy nuts, soy flour, edamame)

Protein Foods to Eat Occasionally

Consider proteins, such as chicken and cheese, condiments rather than main sources of protein. For example, two ounces of chicken or one ounce of blue cheese on a salad, or ricotta cheese topping a taco, is plenty.

- eggs
- poultry (skin removed)
- low-fat dairy products (soft cheeses, cottage cheese, ricotta)
- nonfat or skim milk
- lean red meats
- nut butters, peanut butter, seed butter, legume butters
- skim-milk cheeses (5 grams or less per ounce)
- hard cheeses such as sharp cheese or Parmesan (which has a lot of flavor, so you can use less)
- kidneys
- liver

Protein Foods to Avoid

Try to stay away from these foods altogether.

- pork
- marbled red meats
- salami
- sausage
- smoked meats

Red Meat and the Little People

When we eat red meat, the little people of the intestines get pretty disgusted with the slimy, fatty stuff that coats the walls. They work overtime to clean the fat out of the intestines and send it off to the bloodstream. There it becomes fatty acids and cholesterol. Much of the cholesterol cannot be cleaned out of the arteries. It's just too sticky, like tar, and forms a tacky surface on the arterial walls that builds up into plaque, which eventually reduces the blood flow. If the fat can't be used for energy, it will just end up getting packed away in your body's fat cells. Once it's locked up, it's forgotten and generally stays there—in your thighs or tummy—for a long time. For the sake of the little people, make legumes and fish the main sources of protein in your meal plan. Eat poultry, eggs, and cheese in small quantities only.

7

Micronutrients as Metabolic Support

$\mathcal{V}$itamins, minerals, and trace minerals are called **micronu-trients** because they are required only in small amounts com-pared with the macronutrients (carbohydrates, proteins, fat, and water). They are essential components in enzymes and coenzymes. **Enzymes** are important catalysts that trigger meta-bolic chemical reactions.

Vitamins are essential to life. They regulate **metabolism** and assist biochemical processes such as energy release from food in your digestive system. They are the **coenzymes** that activate the enzymatic pathways necessary for all bodily functions. Some of the major vitamins are water soluble; others are soluble in fat.

Minerals and trace minerals are inorganic elements that are necessary for bone and tissue growth, electrical impulses, enzy-matic reactions, proper metabolism, and oxygen distribution, among other functions. They can be obtained through food or supplements.

Supplements

There are many eating habits that create the risk of vitamin and mineral deficiencies. Reduced nutrient content of our food owing to depleted soil, herbicides, pesticides, and alterations through genetic engineering all contribute to the reality that even a whole-foods diet may need to be supplemented with nutrients. Everything we do, from smoking to exercise to sleep-ing patterns, affects our risk for developing vitamin and mineral deficiencies. These physical and psychological stresses increase our need for many micronutrients. Supplementation is often necessary to replenish lost nutrients, especially in the case of blood sugar imbalances.

Supplements and the Little People

Taking a vitamin and mineral supplement is one of the easiest ways to help the little people do their jobs. Taking potassium, for example, affects insulin sensitivity, responsiveness, and secretion. A high potassium intake also helps protect the immune system from heart disease, atherosclerosis, and cancer. Potassium is an important electrolyte that functions as the phone line for the nerve and muscle cells to communicate with each other.

The RDAS (recommended dietary allowances) for vitamins and minerals were developed by the Food and Nutrition Board of the National Research Council. The RDAS are defined as "the levels of intake of essential nutrients that, on the basis of scientific knowledge, are judged by the Food and Nutritional Board to be adequate to meet the known nutrient needs of practically all healthy persons." (You can find RDAS on package labels for food and supplements in the % Daily Value column. See discussion beginning on page 209 of Chapter 16.) Because people with diabetes are at various stages of wellness or illness, the RDAS are only guidelines for the levels of essential nutrients they should be consuming. The current RDAS were designed for the general population, but substantial amounts of research indicate that people with diabetes have an increased need for specific micronutrients. Studies on the major minerals, trace minerals, and vitamins involved in glucose metabolism have highlighted several nutrients as critical players in the origins of type 2 diabetes. (Boyle et al. 1977, Foster 1987)

Micronutrients (vitamins and minerals) that are especially important in aiding blood sugar regulation are found in whole plant foods. Whole foods are rich in inositol, pyridoxine, niacin, vitamin B_{12}, vitamin C, phosphorus, and nicotinamide, which may reduce such diabetic complications as neuropathy, nephropathy, retinopathy, and microangiopathy. Preliminary tests of supplementation show promise in reducing complications of diabetes. Including these nutrients in your diet may improve your health by inhibiting nonenzymatic protein glycation, inhibiting sorbitol pathway activity by aldose reductase inhibitors, inhibiting the increase in vascular permeability, and preventing oxidative stress and free-radical generation. (Clements 1986, Schatz et al. 1996)

If you have a nutrient deficiency, eating foods rich in the particular nutrient is sometimes enough to bring your level up to normal. But sometimes the deficiency is severe enough to warrant supplementation. In this case, your doctor may prescribe a therapeutic dose for a few weeks and then retest you. When normal, healthy levels are restored, a maintenance dose of that nutrient may be advised to keep the nutrient deficiency from recurring.

Whole foods are always the best source of nutrients, but in the case of diabetes there are such strong correlations between deficiency of specific nutrients and complications that supplements should be used to restore nutrients quickly when a deficiency is diagnosed. In fact, it's a good idea for anyone with diabetes to take a basic multivitamin and mineral complex daily. Just keep in mind that whole foods contain nutrients science hasn't even identified yet, so supplements don't contain them.

If you suspect a nutrient deficiency, increase foods rich in that nutrient in your diet. Ask your diabetes specialist to look for physical signs of deficiency and to perform the appropriate blood test. Use vitamin and mineral supplements when necessary to maintain optimal levels of all nutrients known to regulate blood sugar.

Supplementing Fatty Acids

People with diabetes have impaired metabolism of essential fatty acids (EFAs). Supplementation improves vasodilation nerve conduction and reduces the incidence of microangiopathy and neuropathy. (Cameron et al. 1993) A lack of EFAs in the diet plays a significant role in the development of chronic degenerative diseases such as heart disease, multiple sclerosis, cancer, and rheumatoid arthritis. Experts estimate that 80 percent of Americans do not get enough EFAs.

Essential fatty acids are found in fish oil and flaxseed oil, which provide the linoleic and linolenic acid necessary for the proper development of nerve cells and cellular membranes and production of prostaglandins. Flaxseed oil is inexpensive, widely available, not of animal origin, and the richest source of omega-3 fatty acids known at this time. One tablespoon daily appears to be enough supplementation for those with diabetes.

Fat-Soluble Vitamins and Metabolism

Fat-soluble vitamins are metabolic catalysts that activate the enzymatic pathways in the metabolism of food and its use for energy. Unlike the water-soluble vitamins (discussed later in this chapter), they can be stored in the body's fatty tissue and liver and accumulate over time. The fat-soluble vitamins are A, D, E, and K.

Warning: When supplementing any fat-soluble vitamin or oil, you must also take a vitamin E supplement to protect against oxidation.

Vitamin A (Beta-Carotene)

Beta-carotene is converted to vitamin A in your liver. There are many plant foods rich in beta-carotene to choose from. Because animals eat foods containing beta-carotene and convert the beta-carotene in their livers to vitamin A, animal livers are especially rich in vitamin A. The problem with getting your vitamin A from eating animal livers is that the liver is a filtering organ and may also contain accumulations of pesticides, heavy metals, and other toxic waste. Fish is an excellent source of fat-soluble vitamins. Eat several beta-carotene–rich fruits and vegetables as well as fish daily. Aim for 15,000 international units (IU) a day.

Sources of Beta-Carotene

apricots	peaches
cantaloupe	pumpkin
carrots	red peppers
dandelion greens	spinach
garlic	spirulina
green and yellow vegetables	squash
kale	sweet potatoes
mustard	Swiss chard
papaya	turnip greens
parsley	watercress
	yellow squash

Vitamin D

When you eat foods that contain vitamin D, your liver and kidneys convert it to the active form, which aids in calcium and phosphorus absorption, hair growth, bone and teeth development, osteoporosis prevention, immunity enhancement, and prevention of hypocalcemia (calcium deficiency in the blood).

Vitamin D and calcium should be taken together. Sun on your skin helps your body make vitamin D. It doesn't take a lot of sun to do the job; in fact, just 15 minutes of sunshine daily is enough exposure.

VITAMIN D$_3$

A form of vitamin D called vitamin D$_3$ analog (1 alpha-25-(OH)2-20-epi-22oxa-24,26,27-trishomo-vitamin D) has been used in a trial study to prevent diabetes by restoring suppressor-

---

Sources of Vitamin D

alfalfa	oatmeal
eggs	salmon
fish liver oils	sweet potatoes
halibut	tuna

---

cell activity. (Mathieu et al. 1995) Generally, vitamin D supplements are not fully activated and require conversion by the liver and then by the kidneys. Vitamin D_3 analog appears to be the most easily assimilated form of vitamin D available. The recommended dose is 400 iu per day.

Vitamin E

Studies indicate that people with diabetes benefit from supplementation with vitamin E, which reduces the damage caused by oxidative stress. It also assists insulin uptake, especially among the older population with type 2 diabetes. Vitamin E may help reduce blood pressure and protect kidneys. (Kuznetsov et al. 1994, Gerstein et al. 1996)

Deficiency of the powerful **antioxidant** vitamin E has been found to correlate directly with risk for developing heart disease. (Schleicher et al. 1997, Jain et al. 1996) Diabetes is directly associated with an increased risk of developing premature atherosclerosis, which is thought to be due to high levels of LDLs and their oxidation. Vitamin E's antioxidant potential neutralizes the LDLS.

A study in Italy in 1993 showed vitamin E supplementation resulted in small but significant improvement with control of type 2 diabetes. Studies by Paolisso and colleagues in 1993 also found that vitamin E improved insulin action. Recent studies have shown that even a moderate dose (100 iu a day) can significantly lower glycosylated hemoglobin and triglyceride levels. (Jain et al. 1996)

General biological effects include antioxidant action, circulation improvement, tissue repair, reduction of blood clotting, scar reduction, blood pressure maintenance, cataract prevention, and age-spot prevention. Take 100 to 400 IU a day.

Sources of Vitamin E

brown rice	oatmeal
cold-pressed vegetable oils	seeds
dark-green leafy vegetables	wheat germ
dry beans	wheat germ oil
legumes	whole-grain cereals
nuts	

Vitamin K

Vitamin K plays an important role in the conversion of glucose into glycogen for storage in the liver. Vitamin K is also needed for blood clotting, bone formation and osteoporosis prevention, and regulation of blood pressure. The recommended dose is 100 micrograms a day.

Sources of Vitamin K

broccoli	safflower oil
brussels sprouts	soybeans
cabbage	steel-cut oats
cauliflower	wheat
dark-green leafy vegetables	whole grains

Gamma Linolenic Acid (GLA)

GLA is an antioxidant that plays a special function in the regulation of the immune defense cells known as the T lymphocytes. Your body converts GLA from vegetable oils with the assistance of zinc, magnesium, vitamin C, pyridoxine, niacin, and vitamin A. Deficiencies in any of these nutrients or too much high-fat food, specifically hydrogenated oils such as margarine, may interfere with the conversion of GLA.

Although it is possible (and popular right now) to supplement with evening primrose oil, the omega-3 oils, black currant seed and borage oil are more efficient. Research shows that GLA supplementation decreases tissue EPA. Flaxseed oil is the highest-quality source of EPA. It is an inexpensive source of linoleic acid and contains more than twice as much omega-3 as fish oil. Supplementing with omega-3 oils decreases inflammatory leukotrienes and increases necessary prostaglandin production.

General biological functions include maintaining heart rate, proper vascular dilation, fat metabolism, and blood clotting as well as helping protect against diabetic nerve disease. The recommended dose is 240–480 milligrams per day.

Sources of GLA

black currant seed oil	fish and fish oils
borage oil	flaxseeds and flaxseed oil

Water-Soluble Vitamins

Water-soluble vitamins must be taken in daily, from food or supplements, because they cannot be stored in the body. They are absorbed and used, then excreted in one hour to four days. They include the B vitamins, vitamin C, and the bioflavonoids.

The B vitamins help to maintain nerve conduction; healthy skin, eyes, hair, mouth, and liver; and muscle tone in the gastrointestinal tract. Most of the B vitamins function as parts of enzymes. They work synergistically, which means they should be taken together. This is why the supplement is sold as a B complex. Always take a B vitamin with food to avoid stomach irritation. Do not buy a time-release supplement, because each vitamin is absorbed in a different area of the GI tract. The vitamins released past their absorption point will be lost in the feces.

The B vitamins are thiamine (B_1), riboflavin (B_2), niacin (B_3), pantothenic acid (B_5), pyroxidine (B_6), cobalamin (B_{12}), and folic acid. Biotin, carnitine, choline, and inositol are related to vitamin B.

Vitamin C is an antioxidant that also helps you metabolize sugar and fat. The bioflavonoids enhance absorption of vitamin C. They include rutin, hesperetin, hesperidin, and quercetin, among others. Although they are not true vitamins, their activity is similar, so they are discussed briefly in this section. So is Coenzyme Q_{10}, a bioenzyme.

Vitamin B₁ (Thiamine)

Thiamine deficiency results in impaired mental function and is implicated in neuropathy. Thiamine is occasionally low in people with diabetes. To correct a possible deficiency, take a multivitamin that includes thiamine. Thiamine enhances circulation, hydrochloric acid production, blood formation, and carbohydrate metabolism. A supplemental dose of 50 to 100 milligrams per day, along with a B vitamin complex, is recommended.

The active form of thiamine is *thiamine diphosphate* (TDP). It is the **cofactor** needed for the enzyme system essential to produce energy, synthesize lipids, and manufacture the neuro-

Sources of Thiamine

asparagus	peanuts
beans	peas
broccoli	rice bran
brussels sprouts	soybeans
cut oats	wheat germ
nuts	whole grains

transmitter acetylcholine. Acetylcholine is involved in muscle tone and nerve maintenance and conduction. Thiamine is lost when grains are refined.

The Energy Releasers

Thiamine (B_1), riboflavin (B_2), niacin (B_3), and pantothenic acid (B_5) are all involved in energy production through the citric acid cycle. Without adequate amounts of these water-soluble vitamins, energy could not be freed from storage in the carbohydrate bonds. Among the most important functions of the B vitamins are their roles in enzyme systems. The active forms of most of the B vitamins are coenzymes, the parts of enzymes that cannot be manufactured by the body and so must be obtained from food. Before a vitamin can work as part of an enzyme, it must first be converted into its active coenzyme form.

Vitamin B_2 (Riboflavin)

People with diabetes appear to metabolize riboflavin abnormally. Riboflavin-5-phosphate (R5P) is the most effective form of supplemental riboflavin for them. (Kodentsova et al. 1993, 1994) It's a macronutrient metabolism catalyst that also helps vitamin A heal the lining of the digestive tract and aids in the metabolism of tryptophan. The recommended supplemental dose is five to ten milligrams a day in the R5P form.

Most riboflavin is found naturally as two flavocoenzymes: flavin mononucleotide (FMN) and flavin adenine dinucleotide (FAD). Enriched foods and vitamins supply riboflavin in its free form. In the brush border of the intestine, FMN and FAD are converted into free riboflavin for absorption, bound to plasma proteins for transport, and then carried to the liver for conversion back into FMN and FAD. These two coenzymes are necessary for energy production. Riboflavin is necessary for the conversion of tryptophan to niacin (vitamin B_3). It also aids in converting folacin to its active form and pyridoxine (B_6) to its active form.

The need for riboflavin increases with energy intake and growth needs. Thyroid hormones and adrenal steroids enhance the production of FAD and FMN; tricyclic antidepressants and phenothiazines inhibit their production. If you supplement your diet with fiber supplements or laxatives made of psyllium seed, you may need more riboflavin because this fiber may bind riboflavin.

Sources of Riboflavin

asparagus	currant berries
avocados	fish
beans	nuts
broccoli	spinach
brussels sprouts	yogurt

Vitamin B₃ (Niacin)

Niacin is involved in the regulation of blood sugar, antioxidant mechanisms, and detoxification reactions. Supplementation helps regulate high cholesterol levels. *Niacin*, the nicotinic acid or nicotinate form, is an effective reducer of blood cholesterol. *Niacinamide*, the nicotinamide form, is useful in arthritis treatment and early-onset type 1 diabetes.

In doses of fifty milligrams or more, niacin typically causes skin flushing. To avoid this, the industry has produced a time-release formula—which unfortunately can cause liver damage. An alternative is the hexanicotinate form, which has been used safely in Europe for more than thirty years.

Niacin is an integral part of the enzymes that play important roles in metabolizing fat, cholesterol, and carbohydrate. Niacinamide deficiency causes impaired production of adrenal and sex hormones.

Nicotinamide is a specific form of vitamin B₃ that protects beta cells from autoimmune destruction. High doses of niacinamide have halted the destruction of beta cells in animal studies. Several studies have examined nicotinamide's mechanisms for preventing beta-cell damage. (Karjalainen et al. 1992, Gale 1996, Pozzilli et al. 1996, Taboga et al. 1994) They found that although niacinamide has the greatest effect on diabetes in the phase when beta cells are being destroyed, this is generally the phase that goes unnoticed, before diagnosis. So people who are genetically predisposed to diabetes might take a nicotinamide supplement to reduce their chance of developing the disease.

Niacin is the generic word for *nicotinic acid* and its derivatives, the niacin*amides* (*nicotinamide* and *nicotinic acid amide*). Niacin is absorbed in the stomach and small intestine. It is believed to be converted by the mucosal cells into nicotinamide, the form in which it circulates in the blood. Nicotinamide is an essential component of *nicotinamide adenine dinucleotide* (NAD) and *nicotinamide adenine dinucleotide phosphate* (NADP), coenzymes needed for energy production, fatty-acid synthesis, and protein metabolism. Niacin is part of *glucose tolerance factor* (GTF), the complex essential for glucose regulation, and is essential for the synthesis of various hormones, including insulin.

Niacin is obtained through the diet but can also be manufactured by the body from the amino acid tryptophan. Up to half of the RDA can be obtained this way. Conversion of tryptophan to niacin requires three other B vitamins: thiamine, riboflavin, and pyridoxine.

Niacin is more stable than the other B vitamins and resists heat, light, acid, alkali, and oxidation, so little is lost to food preparation and cooking. The recommended dose is twenty milligrams a day.

Niacinamide is an immunosuppressive drug used to keep type 2 diabetes from progressing to type 1. Drugs are often used after initial diagnosis to suppress the body's immune response to the beta cells, but this treatment is generally effective for only about a year before the patient must take insulin. Niacinamide has been used during this period with similar results and appears to be a safer alternative to drugs than immunosuppressive agents. (Vague et al. 1989, Schmerthaner 1995). Niacinamide improves circulation, nervous system function, macronutrient metabolism, and hydrochloric acid production and reduces cholesterol. The supplemental dose is one to three grams per day.

Sources of Niacin

broccoli	tomatoes
fish	whole wheat
potatoes	

Vitamin B₅ (Pantothenic Acid)

Vitamin B_5 (Pantothenic Acid)

Vitamin B_5 is an important cofactor in lipid metabolism and cholesterol maintenance. Supplementing your diet with fresh garlic is an effective treatment for elevated cholesterol. Dried garlic capsules like Kyolic can also be used. Vitamin B_5 has been shown to lower blood lipids in people with diabetes and reduce the deterioration caused by neuropathy. It is integral to antibody formation, vitamin utilization, macronutrient metabolism, and adrenal support.

Pantothenic acid is obtained from food as part of Coenzyme A (CoA). During digestion, the pantothenic acid is released from the coenzyme and absorbed into the cell, where it is resynthesized into CoA.

As part of Coenzyme A, pantothenic acid is involved in not only the release of energy from carbohydrate but also energy formation from fat and protein, the breakdown and use of fatty acids, and the synthesis of some neurotransmitters, such as acetylcholine. Milling cereal grains reduces their content of pantothenic acid by 50 percent.

Pantothenic acid supplements can be taken in therapeutic doses of 200 to 300 milligrams three times a day or a maintenance dose of 100 milligrams daily.

Sources of Pantothenic Acid

beans	rye bread
bran cereal	saltwater fish
fresh vegetables	whole grains

Vitamin B₆ (Pyridoxine)

Preliminary studies have found that people with diabetes and neuropathy generally have a pyridoxine deficiency. In one study, supplementation of fifty milligrams of pyridoxine reduced the symptoms of retinopathy and reduced pain within ten days. (Jones and Gonzales 1978) Although patients with a pyridoxine deficiency showed marked improvement, those who were not deficient at the onset of supplementation did not benefit from treatment. (Ellis et al. 1991, Hollenbeck et al. 1983, Jones and Gonzales 1978, Kodentsova et al. 1993, Rieder et al. 1980) Correcting a deficiency can correct neuropathy, retinopathy, and damagingly high homocysteine levels. Pyridoxine inhibits the formation of homocysteine, which attacks the heart muscle and allows cholesterol to deposit. People with diabetes who suffer from neuropathy should also be aware of the benefit from supplementing inositol (discussed later in this section).

Vitamin B₆ helps in hydrochloric acid function, fat and protein metabolism, electrolyte balance, red blood–cell formation, nervous system function, brain function, immune system function, antibody production, and hormone production. It also helps the body absorb B₁₂. Supplementation of B₆ may prevent other diabetic complications because it inhibits glycosylation of proteins. (Solomon and Cohen 1989)

A supplement of pyridoxine can be taken in a therapeutic dose of 150 milligrams a day and a maintenance dose of 50 to 100 milligrams a day. For those with peripheral nerve damage, the recommended dosage is 150 milligrams a day.

Sources of Pyridoxine

avocados	peas
bananas	salmon
beans	spinach
brewer's yeast	sunflower seeds
cabbage	walnuts
fish	wheat germ
nuts	whole grains

Vitamin B$_{12}$ (Cobalamin)

Vitamin B$_{12}$, or cobalamin, is occasionally low in people with diabetes. Vitamin B$_{12}$ aids in formation of red blood cells, antibody production, cell respiration and growth, treatment for cataracts, iron absorption, and vitamin B$_6$ absorption. It is needed for the development of the neurotransmitter acetylcholine and it is used in the treatment of diabetic neuropathy.

Sources of Cobalamin

clams	mackerel
herring	nutritional yeast
kidneys	seafood
liver	

Nutritional yeast, fermented soy products (such as miso and tempeh), and seafood are the best sources of B$_{12}$ for people with diabetes.

The treatment dose, in the form of methylcobalamin (active B$_{12}$), is 1,000 micrograms daily. The maintenance dose is 300 micrograms daily.

Folic Acid

Folic acid should be taken with a vitamin B complex. Take a high-quality multivitamin that contains folic acid, B_6, and B_{12} in combination because all three play important roles in homocysteine reduction. Elevated homocysteine levels are a known risk factor in heart disease. It is estimated that 400 micrograms of folic acid daily could reduce the number of heart attacks in Americans by 10 percent.

Folic acid aids in energy production, red blood–cell formation, DNA synthesis, cell division, and protein metabolism. The maintenance dose is 400 micrograms a day.

Sources of Folic Acid

barley	root vegetables
beans	salmon
bran	tuna
brewer's yeast	split peas
green leafy vegetables	wheat germ
lentils	whole grains
	yeast

Biotin

Biotin supplementation has been shown to increase both insulin sensitivity and the activity of the enzyme glucokinase, which is generally low in people with diabetes. (Reddi et al. 1988) Glucokinase is necessary for proper glucose metabolism in the liver, so high doses of biotin improve glucose metabolism.

One study showed that supplementation of sixteen milligrams of biotin per day significantly lowered fasting blood sugar levels. (Coggeshall et al. 1985) In a study of type 2 diabetes, similar effects were noted with nine milligrams of biotin per day. (Zhang et al. 1996) High-dose biotin supplementation has also been an effective treatment in severe diabetic neuropathy.

(Koutsikos et al. 1990) Biotin plays many important roles, including aiding in macronutrient metabolism, cell growth, fatty-acid production, and absorption of the B vitamins. It reduces sugar cravings, prevents hair loss, maintains healthy sweat glands, helps normal nerve tissue and bone marrow develop, and enhances glucose utilization.

A biotin deficiency is rare because biotin can be produced in the intestines from foods. But eating raw egg whites may cause a biotin deficiency. They contain a protein called ovidin, which combines with biotin in the intestinal tract and inhibits proper absorption.

The dosage for deficiency is 1,000 micrograms three times a day. The maintenance dose is 300 micrograms daily.

Sources of Biotin	
brewer's yeast	soybeans
rice bran	soy flour
rice germ	walnuts
saltwater fish	whole grains

Carnitine

Some studies have found people with diabetes to have low carnitine levels. (Cederblad et al. 1982) Carnitine deficiency leads to impaired fat metabolism. Experts recommend supplements for diabetics who have a predisposition to cardiovascular disease as well as reduced kidney and liver function. Carnitine has been shown to greatly improve diabetic vascular and nerve function. (Greco et al. 1992)

Blood plasma tests are recommended when a deficiency is suspected. Red meat and dairy products contain carnitine, but for the most part they do not belong in the diabetic diet. So supplementation in the form of L-carnitine is recommended if a deficiency is diagnosed. The dose is 1,500 milligrams a day.

Sources of Carnitine

dairy	meat
fish	yogurt

Choline

Choline helps the liver release glycogen, minimizes excess fat in the liver, aids in hormone production, and is an integral part of fat and cholesterol metabolism. Choline functions in nerve transmission, gallbladder regulation, and lecithin formation. Choline deficiency can lead to impaired memory and brain function. The recommended dose is 100 milligrams a day.

Sources of Choline

brussels sprouts	pecans
kale	spinach
peanuts	trout
	wheat germ

Inositol

Inositol supplementation is an effective treatment for diabetic neuropathy, a nerve disease caused by diabetes. Inositol deficiency decreases nerve function. (Gregersen et al. 1983) Inositol supports hair growth, prevents hardening of the arteries, aids in lecithin formation, is necessary for cholesterol metabolism, and helps remove fats from the liver.

Supplementation of 1,000 to 2,000 milligrams to restore intracellular inositol levels has been known to reverse diabetic neuropathy. This treatment dose is taken in 500 milligrams two to three times a day. The maintenance dose is 100 milligrams a day. There are no known side effects but there must be methyl donors, like choline and folic acid, available for the inositol to work. Taking a multivitamin will provide all of these nutrients in their symbiotic doses.

Sources of Inositol

citrus fruits	seeds
legumes	whole grains
nuts	

Vitamin C (Ascorbic Acid)

Preliminary studies with type 2 diabetes show that vitamin C aids in sugar and fat metabolism. (Paolisso 1995) Most importantly, vitamin C is a powerful antioxidant; it dramatically reduces free-radical damage. Oxidative stress plays a role in the development of long-term diabetic late complications. Insulin facilitates the transport of this free-radical scavenger into cells, where it neutralizes free-floating electrons so they can't damage blood vessels. Because diabetes is associated with increased free-radical damage to blood vessels and eyes, this is of particular concern. (Sinclair et al. 1994)

Vitamin C is also important in manufacturing the protein substance *collagen*. Collagen is the building material for such tissues as connective tissue, cartilage, and tendons. Vitamin C deficiency leads to poor wound healing, bleeding gums, easy bruising, susceptibility to infection, elevated cholesterol levels, a depressed immune system, increased capillary permeability, and depression. Vitamin C is also necessary for a healthy immune system, proper development of hormones (such as insulin), and the absorption of other nutrients.

Other benefits of vitamin C supplementation for diabetes include reduction of sorbitol accumulation within the cells, improvement in blood sugar control, and inhibition in the glycosylation of proteins.

A powdered, buffered vitamin C supplement gives you the advantage of slower absorption and quantity control. The term *buffered* simply means that calcium and magnesium have been added to the product to slow the uptake and give longer-lasting effects. The powdered form lets you measure exactly how much you'd like to take. This is helpful, as you may want to take more when you are sick or not eating well and less when you are eating foods rich in vitamin C. If you experience gas or loose stools, you have hit the maximum amount your body can absorb. This is called reaching your "bowel tolerance" level for vitamin C. If you have these symptoms, simply cut back the amount you're taking.

Vitamin C is water soluble and is eliminated from the body within twelve hours, even in large doses. Buffered vitamin C breaks down more slowly and extends the amount of time your body will benefit from its release up to sixteen hours. But for optimal absorption, take smaller doses throughout the day. Do not take oral hypoglycemic agents like Diabinase (or any oral medications) at the same time of day as vitamin C. The suggested daily dose for those with diabetes is 1,000 to 3,000 milligrams total daily, in divided doses (three times a day).

THE GLYCOSYLATION PROBLEM

When sugars in the bloodstream bind with proteins, it is known as *glycosylation*. This can dramatically change the structure and function of body proteins. In diabetes, glycosylation of the blood protein albumin results in damage to the corneal lens of the eye and the myelin sheath of nerves. Glycosylated LDL molecules (found in high levels in people with diabetes) do not bind to LDL receptors or shut off cholesterol synthesis in the liver. Therefore, diabetics often have elevated cholesterol levels and an increased risk of atherosclerosis. Fortunately, 1,000 to 3,000 milligrams of vitamin C daily has a tremendous effect in reducing their glycosylation of proteins.

Bioflavonoids

Bioflavonoids (also called simply flavonoids) enhance absorption of vitamin C and should be taken with it. There are many bioflavonoids, including rutin, hesperetin, hesperidin, and quercetin. They are not made by the body and must be taken in through food or supplements. Bioflavonoids promote circulation

Sources of Vitamin C

asparagus	lemons
avocados	mustard greens
beet greens	onions
berries	papaya
broccoli	parsley
brussels sprouts	persimmons
cabbage	radishes
cantaloupe	rose hips
cauliflower	spinach
citrus fruits	strawberries
collard greens	sweet bell peppers
currants	Swiss chard
grapefruit	tomatoes
green leafy vegetables	turnip greens
kale	watercress

and relieve pain, swelling, and bruising. They also stimulate bile production, protect blood vessels, prevent and treat cataracts, and have antibacterial action.

Sources of Bioflavonoids

apricots	leafy greens
black currants	legumes
blue-green algae	lemons
buckwheat	onions
cherries	oranges
citrus peel (the white pithy part)	parsley
grapefruit	rose hips
green tea	

Citrus fruits are a rich source of bioflavonoids. Peel off the outer (colored) layer of the citrus fruit, leaving as much of the white material as possible. Eat the fruit with the white material.

RUTIN

Rutin is a flavonoid responsible for repairing capillary damage. High blood sugar levels over a long period of time stress the integrity of the retina and nerve tissues. Rutin should be taken in a multivitamin to protect against damage. Rutin protects against capillary permeability, bruising, hemorrhoids, and varicose veins. The therapeutic dose is 500 milligrams per day and the maintenance dose is 150 to 200 milligrams per day.

Sources of Rutin

berries	legumes
citrus fruits (the white	onions
pithy part of the peel)	parsley
green tea	

Coenzyme Q₁₀

The bioenzyme Coenzyme Q_{10} (CoQ_{10}) is a vitaminlike substance that resembles vitamin E. Also known as ubiquinone, it is a very potent antioxidant. Studies have shown that people with diabetes have a greater incidence of CoQ_{10} deficiency than those without it. Supplementation has reduced fasting blood sugar levels and ketone bodies. (Kishi et al. 1976, Shigeta et al. 1966)

CoQ_{10} levels decline with age, so a lack of it may contribute to aging. CoQ_{10} supplementation has been used successfully in Japan to treat heart disease and high blood pressure and to enhance the immune system. Other studies show improvement of allergies, asthma, neuropathy, and mental function in schizophrenia and Alzheimer's disease. Supplementation has been helpful for patients with diabetes mellitus, cardiovascular disease, congestive heart failure, high blood pressure, cardiomyopathy, mitral valve prolapse, angina, periodontal disease, immune deficiency, cancer, weight loss, and muscular dystrophy, as well as those who have had coronary artery bypass surgery. For more information on CoQ_{10}'s effects for these conditions, see *The Encyclopedia of Nutritional Supplements* by Michael T. Murray, N.D. (Prima Publishing).

All plant foods contain some CoQ_{10}, but in insignificant quantities. Therefore, diabetics need to take CoQ_{10} supplements. The therapeutic dose is 120 milligrams a day.

Minerals and Trace Minerals

Minerals and trace minerals play key roles in metabolizing blood sugar. Eating foods rich in these nutrients will help reduce the incidence of deficiencies and aid in blood sugar maintenance. Among the most important of these minerals are chromium, copper, manganese, magnesium, potassium, selenium, vanadium, and zinc.

Chromium

Chromium is a trace mineral that is part of the niacin-containing glucose tolerance factor (GTF). GTF works with insulin to make sure it is absorbed and used by your cells so that glucose levels in the blood remain even.

It is estimated that one-quarter to one-half of Americans are deficient in this mineral. Refined diets high in fat and white sugar are inherently low in chromium. Such diets also increase the need for chromium and cause more chromium to be excreted. The lack of chromium in our soil and water supply, plus a diet of refined flour, white sugar, and refined foods, put many of us at risk of chromium deficiency.

Some researchers believe that two out of three Americans have hypoglycemia, prehypoglycemia, or diabetes. Chromium deficiency is so common in people who develop blood sugar disorders or obesity that scientists now consider chromium deficiency a causative factor in the development of diabetes. (Mertz 1993, Mooradian et al. 1994)

GTF is needed for energy metabolism. Chromium is the key mineral in glucose metabolism. It unlocks the cells to allow insulin to carry sugar out of the blood and into the cells. Without enough chromium, insulin cannot carry glucose into the cells. When glucose is blocked from uptake, it builds up in the blood, resulting in high blood sugar. Chromium increases the number of insulin receptors on red blood cells and insulin sensitivity, which can help stabilize blood sugar levels by reducing fasting glucose levels, improving glucose tolerance, and lowering blood insulin levels. Chromium also enhances insulin binding and reduces overall insulin requirements.

People with a chromium deficiency may find that taking a supplement reduces their blood sugar levels immediately. Chromium supplementation has been used effectively for many primary and peripheral disorders of diabetes and hypoglycemia.

Chromium is vital for proper synthesis of fat, cholesterol, and protein. It plays a role in fat metabolism by regulating blood cholesterol levels. Patients with advanced heart disease often have low chromium levels in their blood. Supplementing the diet with chromium has been shown to decrease total cholesterol and triglyceride levels while increasing HDL levels. Several recent studies show that people who supplement with chromium lose weight while increasing lean body mass. Supplementation often reverses the deficiency conditions related to type 2 diabetes. It decreases fasting glucose levels, improves glucose tolerance, and lowers insulin levels. (Abraham et al. 1992, Mossop 1983, Rabinowitz et al. 1983)

The forms that physicians are recommending today are polynicotinate and chromium picolinate. Research is advancing quickly in this area, so this may change. The dose for blood sugar regulation is 500 to 1,000 micrograms per day and the therapeutic dose is 200 to 300 micrograms three times a day. People who follow a chromium-rich diet can maintain with 200 to 400 micrograms once a day.

Sources of Chromium

beans	peanut butter
broccoli	rye bread
green peppers	wheat bran
mushrooms	wheat germ
nutritional yeast	whole grains

Copper

Copper is a trace mineral necessary for enzymatic reactions, proper iron and zinc absorption and utilization, collagen production, and bone formation. Copper should be taken as part of a multivitamin because it supports the absorption of other minerals. Copper aids in the synthesis of red blood cells, the formation of elastin (with vitamin C and zinc), taste sensitivity, and hair and skin coloring. In fact, premature graying of the hair can be reversed with a copper supplement when the graying is due to a copper deficiency.

A therapeutic dose for correcting a deficiency is three to five milligrams per day. A maintenance dose is two milligrams per day.

Sources of Copper	
almonds	lentils
avocados	mushrooms
barley	nuts
beans	oats
beet roots	pecans
broccoli	radishes
dandelion greens	salmon
garlic	seafood
green leafy vegetables	shellfish
legumes	soybeans

Manganese

Manganese is an important cofactor in the key enzymes of glucose metabolism. A deficiency can cause diabetes in animals (Nutrition Review 1968) Studies have found that people with diabetes have only half as much manganese as those without it. (Mooradian and Morley 1987) Low manganese levels affect pancreatic tissue integrity; they can directly impair pancreatic insulin synthesis and secretion and increase intracellular insulin degradation.

A deficiency of manganese can lead to glucose intolerance, but supplementation can reverse this effect. One study achieved reversal with only three to five milligrams daily. (Rubinstein et al. 1962, Baldy 1990) Manganese also aids in protein and fat metabolism, nerve function, blood sugar regulation, energy production, bone growth, reproduction, absorption of vitamin E, and metabolism of thiamine. It is essential for treating iron deficiency anemia.

Manganese is taken in a supplemental dose of ten to fifty milligrams per day.

Sources of Manganese

avocados	nuts
blueberries	seaweed
dried peas	seeds
green leafy vegetables	spinach
legumes	whole grains

Magnesium

Magnesium is necessary for the secretion and action of insulin as well as the actions of many enzymes involved in carbohydrate metabolism.

Magnesium levels are low in people with diabetes and lowest in those with severe retinopathy. Magnesium deficiency appears to be a risk factor for the development of retinopathy and cardiovascular disease. (White and Campbell, 1993)

Hyperglycemia, a state caused by uncontrolled diabetes, and insulin injections increase magnesium loss. And the condition of diabetes itself may reduce magnesium levels. Elevated blood sugar levels stimulate excessive urination, which can wash minerals and trace minerals out of the body. When people with insulin-dependent diabetes experience ketoacidosis, there is a marked mineral depletion. In addition, many diabetics take hypertensive medication and/or diuretics. Diuretics cause wasting of all minerals. (Boyle et al. 1977, Mertz 1993, Freund 1979)

The American Diabetes Association (ADA) sponsored a consensus panel to examine these studies. The ADA released its first consensus statement regarding magnesium supplementation in the treatment of diabetes mellitus in 1992. (Anderson 1992). It concluded that serum magnesium affects body magnesium stores. Those taking magnesium supplements have a lower incidence of developing either hypertension or type 2 diabetes.

Supplementation with magnesium may improve insulin response and action. It improves beta-cell response and insulin action in diabetics. (Paolisso et al. 1990) And it may prevent some complications like retinopathy, heart disease, and blood vessel deterioration. (Paolisso and Barbagallo 1997)

People with diabetes need to eat foods rich in magnesium and supplement fifty milligrams of vitamin B_6 (which helps magnesium enter the cell) daily. A supplemental dose is 250 milligrams of magnesium divided into two or three doses daily. A therapeutic dose is 500 milligrams per day. A dose of 400 milligrams per day is recommended for individuals with nonobese diabetes.

Sources of Magnesium

beans	peas
green leafy vegetables	seeds
lentils	tofu
nuts	whole grains

Potassium

People who take insulin injections often have a potassium deficiency. Taking potassium improves insulin sensitivity, responsiveness, and secretion in type 2 diabetes. A supplemental dose of 200 to 500 milligrams a day, along with a diet rich in potassium-containing foods, is recommended.

Sources of Potassium

avocados	peaches
cod	salmon (wild)
flounder	spinach
haddock	tomatoes
lima beans	tuna

Selenium

Selenium is a powerful antioxidant. (Douillet et al. 1996) It offers tremendous benefit in protecting kidneys when taken in combination with vitamin E. The recommended dose is 200 to 400 micrograms a day.

Sources of Selenium

barley	salmon
Brazil nuts	shrimp
haddock	sunflower seeds
lobster	swordfish
oysters	tuna
red Swiss chard	

Vanadium

Vanadium is a trace mineral with no established need in humans, but recent research in humans and animals suggests that it has an insulinlike effect on glucose metabolism. In glucose metabolism studies done in test tubes and on animals, the supplemental form of vanadium, vanadyl sulfate, looks promising in improving oral glucose tolerance. It is thought to produce similar effects in humans. In a human study, supplementation with vanadyl sulfate showed improvement in hepatic and peripheral insulin sensitivity in insulin-resistant type 2 patients. It has also been shown to lower cholesterol levels and blood pressure.

Although how it works is not yet understood, vanadium appears to activate the insulin receptors, increasing the number of glucose transporter proteins in cell membranes. This improves insulin sensitivity. The recommended supplemental dose is 50 to 100 micrograms per day.

Sources of Vanadium

buckwheat	peanut oil
cabbage	safflower oil
oats	soybeans
olive oil	sunflower seeds
parsley	

Zinc

Zinc supplementation may exert insulinlike effects and protect beta cells from oxidative damage. People with diabetes are often found to be deficient in zinc at the time of diagnosis. Deficiency may be more common in diabetics because they excrete increased amounts of zinc in their urine, which lowers their plasma leukocyte and erythrocyte zinc levels.

The RDA for zinc is fifteen milligrams per day. Diabetes exerts a higher degree of metabolic stress, which increases the recommended supplemental dose to thirty milligrams a day taken with copper (to help our bodies absorb the zinc). Zinc is best supplemented as part of a multivitamin and mineral complex.

Supplementing with vanadium and zinc is a prudent part of a supplemental program for people with blood sugar disorders for several reasons. Both vanadium and zinc imitate insulin, thus reducing excessive excretion of insulin and reducing the risk of developing diabetes. (Sprietsma and Schuitemaker 1994) Zinc and vanadium may be depleted from the stress of beta-cell destruction. And low levels of zinc in drinking water have been linked to the development of diabetes. (Haglund et al. 1996).

Supplements of zinc should be taken in a therapeutic dose of thirty milligrams a day with two milligrams of copper or a maintenance dose of fifteen milligrams a day.

Sources of Zinc

almonds	peanuts
Brazil nuts	peas
buckwheat	pecans
gingerroot	pumpkin seeds
green peas	rye
hazelnuts	split peas
lentils	walnuts
lima beans	wheat bran
oats	wheat germ
oysters	whole wheat

Fiber Supplements

Fiber slows the absorption of glucose into the bloodstream, reducing postprandial spikes in blood sugar levels. Taking a fiber supplement daily will help reduce high blood sugar levels. Several studies with fiber and diabetes have found the following results. In one study, sixteen grams of guar gum per day and ten grams of pectin added to a meal containing 106 grams of carbohydrate had significant effects on postprandial blood glucose in type 1 diabetes. Another study found that 4.2 grams of gel fiber in the form of glucomannan added to the diet significantly improved glycemic control, insulin requirement, and HDL cholesterol in those with insulin-dependent diabetes. Taking seven grams of apple pectin ten minutes before a meal decreased insulin required by 35 percent.

If you eat a diet rich in vegetables, beans, peas and lentils, whole grains, and fruit, you will get plenty of fiber. If your diet is not rich in these foods, consider supplementing with fiber pills or powder.

In summary, current research supports the use of a high quality multivitamin and mineral complex for those with blood sugar disorders.

Part II

☙

Meal Plans:
Developing Your
Nutritional Therapy
Regimen

8

The Recording System for Your Individualized Health Program

*E*veryone who has diabetes has a far better chance of living a normal life now and in the future if he or she can keep blood sugar levels between 50 and 150 milliliters per deciliter. However, not everyone with diabetes has the same schedule, habits, personality, knowledge, or resources. Each unique individual will have different preferences and possibilities, particular difficulties, and special situations. This chapter provides some guidance for using an individualized approach that accommodates any number of situations and choices.

The main benefit of this program is that it allows you to keep track of all aspects of your health in one system on a daily basis. With a little effort up front, you can achieve better health.

Achieving better health requires tracking a vast number of facts and figures, such as the following: milligrams of glucose in the blood, cubic centimeters of insulin, milligrams of oral medication, times of day, number of calories, grams of macronutrients (carbohydrate, protein, and fat), tablespoons and ounces of food, pounds of body weight, minutes of exercise, and more.

Because most of us have trouble recalling so many numbers and details, collecting these figures in one place for easy reference is helpful. In this chapter you will find a suggested recording system that provides everything you'll need to schedule, record, observe, analyze, and adjust for continuously better results. It includes the following three parts:

- Blood glucose test recording booklet
- Daily meal plan and health record
- Personal guidelines

Blood Glucose Test Recording Booklet

Ask your doctor, pharmacist, or blood test machine company for this small booklet. It's about the size of your blood-testing machine and has spaces for you to write the type and amount of insulin and/or oral medications and urine ketone test results each time you take them. You will use this daily. Most doctors and nutritionists ask to review these figures periodically.

Daily Meal Plan and Health Record

This part of the recording system consists of one page for each day of the week. Record the following information:
- Types of foods to be eaten for each meal, including portion sizes and number of calories and grams of carbohydrate, protein, and fat.
- Times of day for meals and exercise.
- Symptoms you experience (for example, headaches, stress, menstrual periods, insomnia, extreme thirst, fatigue).
- Suspected causes for extremely high or low blood sugars. Use this daily for as long as you need its support. Some people may outgrow the need for it. Others may alternate its use with periods of "winging it" as they develop new and better habits.

Filling Out Your Daily Meal Plan and Health Record

Choose the Daily Meal Plan and Health Record appropriate to your daily caloric needs (1,500, 2,000, or 2,500 calorie plans) on pages 136–138. If your needs are different than those provided, please refer to the Macronutrient chart on page 133.
1. Enlarge the form and make several photocopies.
2. Using the lines under each mealtime
    - fill in the name of each food item (such as cooked brown rice)

- fill in the quantity of each food item (such as 1 cup or 1 tablespoon)
- fill in the number of grams of carbohydrates, protein, and fats in each serving

(You can find these numbers by reading product labels, using gram counting books, or referring to the nutrition analysis information in a cookbook.)

(To see how this is done, study the sample filled-out form for a 1,500-calorie plan on page 139.)

3. Write the total number of carbohydrates, protein, and fats for each meal.
4. Calculate the number of calories for each meal. The total calories may be calculated this way:
   - multiply the number of grams of carbohydrates $\times$ 4 = number of calories of carbohydrates
   - multiply the number of grams of protein $\times$ 4 = number of calories of protein
   - multiply the number of grams of fat $\times$ 9 = number of calories of fat
5. Record the time(s) you will exercise each day under NOTES.

The Daily Meal and Health Record provides three meals of equal size and one snack that is one-third the size of one meal. You will be aiming for 50 percent carbohydrate, 25 percent protein and 25 percent fat with the day's total caloric intake.

Creating Meals That Fit Your Personal Needs

Find recipes that provide you with all the necessary nutritional information (including total calories, carbohydrates, protein, and fat) as well as serving sizes that fit your plan. When you make up a new recipe, determine the macronutrient breakdown for each ingredient you use. Add up the total and divide it by a number that makes each portion come out closest to what you may eat for one meal. Or simply follow the recipes in *The What to Eat if You Have Diabetes Cookbook* (Contemporary Books, 1999).

Purchase a calorie counter booklet that includes grams of carbohydrates, protein, and fat—as well as portion sizes that are closest to the amount you usually eat, if possible. Cross-reference between the numbers of calories and grams on your meal plan to make sure they both fit your plan. Train yourself to read the amounts of macronutrients on the label before purchasing any food item. This way you will know whether or not it's going to complement your meal plan. Making these decisions ahead of time will help you create quick but healthful meals.

Make a list of cereals, breads, yogurts, and other common food items that fit your personal meal plan and record the brand names to make it easier the next time you go shopping.

Each time you finish planning a week's worth of meals, make out a grocery list that includes every item you'll need to prepare every meal for that week. You will use up the food by the end of the week and you will know that your food was fresh. And if you stick to your list, there will be no need to buy those tempting extras that can only cause you grief when your sugar level goes out of control.

When mealtime is near and/or you are beginning to feel hungry, you can consult your meal plan to find out exactly what you had planned for that time. You know the groceries are on hand and you have only to put them together and measure according to the specifications you already determined. If you wait until you're really hungry to try to figure out what to have, you're less likely to get the calculation right and it will feel like a lot more work.

After you have developed a set of meals for an entire day, save your work. You may want to make these meals in the future.

Suppose you look at your meal plan and spaghetti is listed for dinner, but you don't feel like having spaghetti that night. Just find a more appealing dinner plan from another day's schedule and have that instead. All dinners are planned to contain the same number of calories and a similar breakdown of macronutrients. If one meal calls for an ingredient that will spoil if not eaten within a week or so, such as cottage cheese or chicken,

Macronutrient Ratios
for Individual Caloric Allowances

Based on 3 equal meals + 1 snack
(50% carbohydrates, 25% protein, 25% fat)

Meals

DAILY CALORIC ALLOWANCE	CALORIES PER MEAL	CARBOHYDRATES		PROTEIN		FAT	
		Calories	Grams	Calories	Grams	Calories	Grams
1,350	405	180	45	90	22	90	10
1,500	450	225	56	112	28	112	12
1,750	525	262	65	131	32	131	14.5
2,000	600	300	75	150	37	150	16
2,250	675	337	84	168	42	168	18.5
2,500	750	375	93	187	46	187	20

Snacks

DAILY CALORIC ALLOWANCE	CALORIES PER MEAL	CARBOHYDRATES		PROTEIN		FAT	
		Calories	Grams	Calories	Grams	Calories	Grams
1,350	135	67	16	33	8	33	3.5
1,500	150	73	19	37	9	37	4
1,750	175	87	21	43	10	43	4.5
2,000	200	100	25	50	12	50	5.5
2,250	225	112	28	56	14	56	6
2,500	250	125	31	62	15	62	6.5

you may want to create another meal with that same ingredient so as to use it all up that same week.

You will probably want to make up next week's meal plans and shopping list a couple of days before you eat your last planned meal so you won't suddenly get caught short of groceries.

Find a convenient place to keep your plan for the current day. Attach it to the refrigerator with a magnet, or keep it in a three-ring binder and place it face up in a handy kitchen drawer.

Equivalent Level Measure and Weights

Learning to measure portions requires knowing the equivalents to convert the different measurement units you see on packaging. Try to memorize the most common unit measurements.

60 drops = 1 teaspoon = 5 grams

1 teaspoon = 5 grams

3 teaspoons = 1 tablespoon = 15 grams

2 tablespoons = 30 grams = 1 ounce (fluid)

4 tablespoons = ¼ cup = 60 grams

8 tablespoons = ½ cup = 120 grams

16 tablespoons = 1 cup = 240 grams = 250 ml. = 8 ounces = ½ pound

2 cups = 1 pint = 480 grams = 500 ml. = 16 ounces (fluid) = 1 pound

4 cups = 2 pints = 1 quart = 1,000 ml. = 1 kg. = 2.2 pounds

4 quarts = 1 gallon

HELPFUL HINTS

- Learn the difference between the amounts for cooked pasta and dry pasta. Use a pasta-measuring ring to measure dry pasta. Add lots of onions and mushrooms to bulk up the sauce.
- Restaurant salad dressing can be very high in sugar and fat. If the server can't tell you the nutrition breakdown, skip it. Take your own dressing in a small plastic container.

- Ask a personal exercise trainer how many calories you'll burn in a half hour of treadmill exercise. Then ask your nutritionist where to add these calories during the day to offset the loss.

Visual Measurements

Measure the foods you eat most often into your dishes at home and pay attention to how high you fill them to make up one cup of cereal or milk. Three ounces of meat or cheese is about the size of a pack of playing cards.

1,500-Calorie Meal Plan

DAILY MEAL PLAN and HEALTH RECORD			Date:	Day:	
Daily Calorie Allowance: 1,500		Calories per meal: 450		Calories per snack: 150	
Goals Per Meal	Carb	Pro	Fat	NOTES	
Percentages	50	25	25		
Calories	225	112	112		
Grams	56	28	12		
BREAKFAST TIME:	Carb	Pro	Fat		
Total Grams					
Total Calories:					
LUNCH TIME:	Carb	Pro	Fat		
Total Grams					
Total Calories:					
DINNER TIME:	Carb	Pro	Fat		
Total Grams					
Total Calories:					
SNACK TIME:	Carb	Pro	Fat		
Calories	73	37	37		
Grams	19	9	4		
Total Grams					
Total Calories:					

2,000-Calorie Meal Plan

DAILY MEAL PLAN and HEALTH RECORD				Date: Day:
Daily Calorie Allowance: 2,000	Calories per meal: 600			Calories per snack: 200
Goals Per Meal	Carb	Pro	Fat	NOTES
Percentages	50	25	25	
Calories	300	150	150	
Grams	75	37	16	
BREAKFAST TIME:	Carb	Pro	Fat	
Total Grams				
Total Calories:				
LUNCH TIME:	Carb	Pro	Fat	
Total Grams				
Total Calories:				
DINNER TIME:	Carb	Pro	Fat	
	100	50	50	
	25	12	5.5	
Total Grams				
Total Calories:				
SNACK TIME:	Carb	Pro	Fat	
Calories	100	50	50	
Grams	25	12	5.5	
Total Grams				
Total Calories:				

2,500-Calorie Meal Plan

DAILY MEAL PLAN and HEALTH RECORD				Date: Day:
Daily Calorie Allowance: 2,500 Calories per meal: 750				Calories per snack: 250
Goals Per Meal	Carb	Pro	Fat	NOTES
Percentages	50	25	25	
Calories	375	187	187	
Grams	93	46	20	
BREAKFAST TIME:	Carb	Pro	Fat	
Total Grams				
Total Calories:				
LUNCH TIME:	Carb	Pro	Fat	
Total Grams				
Total Calories:				
DINNER TIME:	Carb	Pro	Fat	
	125	62	62	
	31	15	6.5	
Total Grams				
Total Calories:				
SNACK TIME:	Carb	Pro	Fat	
Calories	125	62	62	
Grams	31	15	6.5	
Total Grams				
Total Calories:				

Sample Daily Record (1,500 cal/day)

DAILY MEAL PLAN and HEALTH RECORD				Date: 3-25		Day: Thursday
Daily Calorie Allowance: 1,500			Calories per meal: 450			Calories per snack: 150
Goals Per Meal	Carb	Pro	Fat	NOTES		
Percentages	50	25	25			
Calories	225	112	112			
Grams	56	28	12			
BREAKFAST TIME: 7:30	Carb	Pro	Fat			
⅓ cup cooked steelcut oats	27	3.5	2			
¾ cup fat free soy milk	5.5	4.5	0			
1 tsp sucanat + ⅛ pinch stevia	4	0	0			
½ cup plain nonfat yogurt	8	5	0			
10 almonds	0	7	10			
1½ cup strawberries	15	1	0			
Total Grams	59.5	21	12			
Total Calories: 430	238	84	108			
LUNCH TIME: 12:30	Carb	Pro	Fat			
Fish Salad Sandwich						
3 oz cooked fish	0	24	7			
1 cup chopped romaine-onion celery-pickle	2	1	0			
1 Tbs Lite Mayo	4	0	1			
1 slice squeezed lemon	0	0	0			
2 pcs. whole grain bread	40	6	4			
½ cup fresh peach or pear	10	0	0			
Total Grams	56	31	12			
Total Calories: 456	224	124	108			
DINNER TIME: 6:00	Carb	Pro	Fat			
1 cup Rice & Beans Italia	41	12	3			
2 cups tossed green salad	8	0	0			
4 Tbs Green Goddess dressing	2	3	3			
2 Tbs sunflower seeds	6	6	7			
Total Grams	57	21	13			
Total Calories: 429	228	84	117			
SNACK TIME: 10:00	Carb	Pro	Fat			
Calories	73	37	37			
Grams	19	9	4			
3 oz edamame	8	7.5	4			
1 cup strawberries	10	0	0			
2 Tbs nonfat yogurt	2	2	0			
Total Grams	20	9.5	4			
Total Calories: 154	80	38	36			

Personal Guidelines for Better Blood Glucose Control

Now you can use your daily meal plan to discover clues that will help you fine-tune your individualized program.

At the end of each day, look at the glucose levels you have recorded in your blood glucose test recording booklet. Record these figures on your Daily Meal Plan and Health Record.

Suppose you see a blood sugar reading of 325 just before dinner on your daily meal planner. Under NOTES just below lunch and just before dinner, write the number 325. Then put on your detective badge and look carefully at the amounts and types of foods you consumed during or after lunch. Think about the foods already listed on your plan. Was one of the portions too large? Maybe you need to review your measuring tools. Did you experience a great deal of stress during this time? Perhaps you could review some basic stress-relieving techniques. Did you eat the restaurant salad dressing even though the macronutrient content was not available? You may want to take your own next time. Were any foods added spontaneously during that time? Did someone bring cake to the office and tempt you with a piece? If so, perhaps you'll need to eat a smaller portion next time—or save the cake to eat with a meal, which will lower its glycemic index and the risk of high blood sugar.

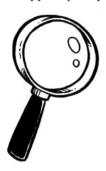

Suppose you spot a blood sugar reading of 45 just before bedtime. Write that number under NOTES just below dinner and before snack. Look at the quantities you ate for dinner or lunch. Did you not finish your meal or forget to eat? Does your blood glucose booklet show that you had to take extra insulin for high blood sugar earlier? Perhaps you took too much. You might want to review your sliding scale for extra insulin with your doctor. Did you exercise too much for the number of calories called for on your meal plan? Write down any clues that you think might explain the discrepancy.

At the end of the week, write out all the clues that you have discovered in list form and call them your personal guidelines for better blood glucose control.

9

Meal Planning

*A*n individual meal plan is based on your blood sugar, cholesterol, and triglyceride levels. Your blood pressure, height, weight, age, medications, and activity level should also be taken into consideration. A nutritionist can help you refine your meal plan. It is helpful to meet with a nutritionist over a period of time so that adjustments can be made when necessary.

Some people with diabetes do not measure or weigh their food and manage to stay healthy. But to do this you would have to eat a much narrower variety of food. For example, when eating out you would want to avoid all sauces and combination foods with unknown quantities of calories and macronutrients. This translates into a lot of plain chicken breasts and refried beans. It's surprising how many hidden calories there are in packaged foods, fast foods, and restaurant fare.

GENERAL RULES
- Distribute calories throughout the day.
- Do not skip meals.
- Take medications at the same time each day.
- Lose weight if necessary.
- Drink at least 32 ounces of purified water daily.
- Eat a variety of fresh, high-quality foods.
- Avoid too much overall fat in your meal plan, particularly saturated fat and cholesterol.
- Eat lots of fiber-rich foods such as beans, peas, lentils, and whole grains. They'll carry your blood sugar longer, which means less insulin and less worry about hypoglycemic reactions.
- Eat minimal amounts of sugar.

- Reduce or eliminate alcohol.
- Quantity is critical; it pays to weigh portions.
- Coordinate food intake with insulin and exercise.

Timing Strategies

Coordinate your food intake with the action of your insulin. Plan to eat meals and snacks according to the levels of insulin being released into your blood. Your diabetes specialist will be able to show you when your insulin is peaking and help you choose mealtimes.

Depending on your medications (insulin, oral hypoglycemic drugs, or no drugs), your nutritionist will help tailor your meal plan to meet your needs.

Insulin acts on the sugar circulating in your blood. That sugar comes from the food you eat or the sugar that is stored in your body, such as glycogen stored in your liver and in your muscles. The key to taking insulin and balancing meals is to match both sides of the equation as closely as possible: sugar in the blood-stream to insulin in the bloodstream.

After all this planning and work, you will

- Feel better and have more energy.
- Reduce your risk of complications.
- Maintain a desirable weight.
- Improve your overall health.

Creating Your Nutritional Needs Profile

To help you clarify what your needs are before going to your first appointment with a dietitian and/or nutritionist, create your specific nutritional needs profile by answering the following questions.

LIFESTYLE
What is your daily work or school schedule?
What is your exercise program?

Do you smoke?
Do you drink alcohol?

MEDICATIONS

Are you taking insulin? If so, how much? What time(s) of day
do you take it? When does it peak?
Are you taking any oral hypoglycemic agents (pills)?
What other medications are you taking?

CURRENT HEALTH

Do you have any other medical conditions that affect your diet?
Do you have other health conditions that affect your activity
level?
Do you have any food allergies or other conditions that affect
your food choices?
Do you have food restrictions due to religious beliefs?

CURRENT DIET

What types of foods do you like?
Do you eat out a lot?
Do you cook much?
Are you a vegetarian?
Are you familiar with whole foods?
Do you generally cook from whole foods (grains, beans, veg-
etables, etc.)?
Do you generally eat packaged foods (canned soups, frozen din-
ners, dried products, boxed cereals, microwave foods, etc.)?

YOUR BODY

What is your height and weight?
What is your healthy weight?
What is your frame size?

CLINICAL DATA

If you have any of this laboratory information from your physician, take it with you to the dietitian or nutritionist.

Do your lab results show protein in your urine?

What are your blood lipid levels?

Do you have records of recent blood sugar tests?

What was the result of your last glycosylated hemoglobin test?

Have you been tested for nutrient deficiencies?

MACRONUTRIENT RATIOS

A fat intake of 25 percent is fairly low compared to the average American diet, but it allows your diet to have a higher percentage of protein and carbohydrates. When your protein and carbohydrate calories come from plant products such as beans, peas, and lentils, the ratio will generally work out to about 50 percent carbohydrate and 25 percent protein. This is ideal, since this portioning of the macronutrients regulates blood sugar.

Carbohydrate   50%
Protein   25%
Fat   25%

Your nutritionist can help you decide the right number of grams of carbohydrates and calories for you. These will be measured amounts of food that contain an average number of grams of carbohydrate, protein, and fat. Each choice provides an average number of calories. The type and number of food choices will depend in part on the number of calories you require to gain, maintain, or lose weight.

Reminder: all this work in calculating your diet will provide greater flexibility in your food choices while meeting the insulin requirements.

Take inventory of your lifestyle and special needs. Write down your questions about how to reach your health goals now that you have diabetes. Meet with a diabetes specialist to set up your individualized plan for medications, exercise, supplements, and nutrition. Keep a record of your goals and your plan for achieving them. Check your notes on a regular basis to be sure you are on track. If your blood sugar is not well controlled, make an appointment with your diabetes specialist to reassess your plan and fine-tune it where needed.

The Underweight Meal Plan

The onset of undiagnosed diabetes can cause wasting of muscle tissue. Insufficiency of insulin results in high blood sugar, which means the food (sugar) is staying in the bloodstream and not getting into the cells to function as energy, make muscle mass, and make fat. Many people who have been newly diagnosed as insulin dependent will need to gain back at least some of that weight. You may be happy to have lost some unwanted fat, but you want to be as close to your ideal body weight (IBW) as possible so that you have enough muscle to be active, keep your back healthy, and feel strong.

Rapid Weight Loss

Very rapid weight loss can result in substantial loss of protein tissue and dehydration. Replacement of lost fluid is crucial to all of your biochemical processes. Approximately 50 to 60 percent of a healthy adult is fluid. Drinking plenty of purified water is the first step in rehydration. Drink an eight-ounce glass of water every hour until you are rehydrated. Then drink one eight-ounce glass of water every two hours for maintenance. The next step is to be sure you have enough available electrolytes for your body to absorb the water properly. Electrolytes are the minerals sodium, potassium, magnesium, calcium, and chloride, which are found naturally in all fruits and vegetables. If you are eating fresh fruits and/or vegetables with each meal, you are getting plenty of electrolytes for proper absorption of water.

To find out if you are underweight, you must first determine your ideal body weight. These numbers will give you a general idea of your target weight. However, many factors are individual, such as bone size and activity level. Those who are very active or athletic will have more muscle mass. Because muscle is heavier than fat, you may weigh more than your IBW and still be very healthy. Or you can be at your IBW according to the chart and still have too much fat and too little muscle.

Even when you are underweight, you can be "overfat." There are tools that measure body fat. Dietitians often use calipers that pinch fat at various places on your body. The measurements are averaged to come up with your overall body-fat percentage. Computerized body-fat calculators, available through sports medicine clinics and high-tech home equipment catalogs, are slightly more accurate than calipers. The most accurate body-fat testing to date is the water immersion tank. Many sports medicine clinics and hospitals and some health clubs have this expensive equipment. Most of us don't need to know our exact body fat, but if you are not gaining weight because you are afraid to gain fat, a body-fat test could help you feel comfortable gaining weight and in control of the process.

Keep in mind that your goal is to gain muscle mass, not fat. Most people find it easy to gain fat—they just sit around watching TV and munching high-calorie snacks like chips, candy, ice cream, and cookies. But if you follow these simple rules, you'll gain muscle as you gain weight.

- Exercise daily. Be active.
- Increase overall food portions, not specific foods.
- Take a basic vitamin and mineral supplement.
- Drink one eight-ounce glass of water every hour.

The overall goal of dietary management is to reduce body fat to improve health and reduce complications while maintaining muscle mass. Important clinical indicators such as plasma glucose, lipids, and blood pressure will determine your individual goals. These goals will be supported when you and your nutritionist design a meal plan made up of foods that you like and want to eat on a regular basis. Keeping a food record for a few days before you meet with the nutritionist will help you identify where you need support.

Identifying Nutrient Deficiencies and Food Allergies

The Daily Meal Plan and Health Record is a useful tool for identifying which types of foods you may be lacking and any food allergies you may have developed. Your nutritionist or dietitian is the part of your medical team who can provide the tools you need to make the changes in your diet. If food allergies are suspected, he or she will also help you find nonallergenic alternative food choices. This person will provide recipes and alternatives, as well as expert private tutoring in the mystifying world of label reading. (See Chapter 16 on reading labels.)

By following the basic diet for regulating blood sugar, you will be eating the right foods for weight gain as well as natural nutrient supplementation. The foods that make up this diet are inherently nutrient rich. A diet high in plant fibers and low in animal products is ideal for gaining muscle weight.

Your dietitian or nutritionist will help you identify the food habits that may be keeping you from gaining the weight you'd like. Your physician will help you determine any medical condition that may be interfering with digestion or metabolism of your food.

Supplements

If you have lost considerable weight, you may have developed nutritional deficiencies. Your nutritionist should be able to identify deficiencies by looking for physical signs and using blood tests. If deficiencies are determined, a high-quality multivitamin can raise nutrient levels. We recommend Thorne Research's Basic Nutrients III or Basic Nutrients IV multivitamin and mineral supplements.

Eat More

It's very simple to increase your overall calories on this program. Stay with the same blood sugar–regulating diet and increase overall calories. Your nutritionist will calculate the number of calories by which to increase your daily diet depending on the number of pounds you need to gain. For example, you may increase from 1,500 calories a day to 2,000 calories. You may eat two slices of toast in the morning rather than just one, but you will still be eating from the same diet. It will keep you on track with carbohydrate, protein, and fat ratios as well as keeping blood lipid and cholesterol levels down. By staying within the basic dietary program, you should be able to control blood sugar levels while gaining muscle mass.

The Overweight Meal Plan

It is critical for people with diabetes who are overweight to get down to and maintain their ideal body weight. Obesity aggravates cardiovascular problems and creates insulin resistance, which raises blood sugar levels. As you lose weight, you will see dramatic improvements in triglyceride levels, blood pressure, and blood sugar levels.

By following the basic meal plan, you will be eating the right foods for weight loss. A meal plan high in plant fibers and low in animal products is ideal for losing weight as well as regulating blood sugar.

Fat Leads to Ineffective Insulin Absorption

Insulin resistance develops from an increase in fat cells. The number of insulin receptor sites located on the surface of the cells decreases in the obese person. The insulin cannot attach to the receptor and therefore cannot deliver the glucose into the cell.

If you are obese (defined as 20 percent or more over your ideal body weight), you will need to make an appointment with a nutritionist. The overall goal of meal planning is to reduce body fat and improve health and reduce complications. Important clinical indicators such as plasma glucose, lipids, and blood pressure will determine your individual goals. These goals will be supported when you and your nutritionist design a meal plan made up of foods that you like and want to eat on a regular basis. Keeping a food record for a few days before you go to your appointment will help you identify where you need support.

Height-weight charts should be used simply as reference points. Many factors affect an individual's ideal body weight, among them family history, athletic history, current activity, fat distribution, complications, and associated conditions. Your nutritionist will take all of this into consideration when determining your individual IBW.

Heavy Habits

Your nutritionist will help you identify the food habits that may be keeping you from losing the weight you'd like to drop. When embarking on a weight-loss path, I find it easier to add in the new healthy choices first; they will nudge out the fat- and sugar-laden foods. Then start to refine your meal plan. Identify your fattening daily habits and work to change them.

Here are some suggestions for breaking a few of the common habits that feed the fat.

- If you drink sodas often, replace them with a sparkling (no-calorie) water like Talking Rain™ (naturally flavored waters).
- If you drink a latte everyday, try a low-fat dairy or low-fat soy-milk latte instead.
- Make a new rule that you won't eat while watching TV. It's easy to forget how much you are eating if you eat out of the bag or the box while watching TV.
- Measure out your portion of crackers or popcorn and put it in a separate bowl. Then put the bag away so you won't eat more than you intended.

- Try the low-cal, no-fat salad dressings or squeeze fresh lemon juice and sprinkle a little sea salt on your salad instead.
- Skip the chips and dip. Instead, try the Japanese appetizer edamame, which is steamed green soybean pods. See the edamame recipe in Chapter 4.
- Opt for nonfat dairy or low-fat soy milk. Use cheese in small quantities only, as you would use a condiment.
- Avoid lard- and butter-based sauces and gravies. Try instead tomato-based pasta sauces, low-calorie broth-based gravies, and tofu or soy-milk cream dressings.

Maintaining your ideal body weight is a critical part of the equation in managing your blood sugar. People with type 1 diabetes must keep their weight down so the insulin injections will work properly. Those with type 2 may be able to control the disease altogether by losing weight.

The Exchange System

The exchange system is outmoded in that it does not take into consideration the benefits of legumes and unprocessed foods. Many people also find the system is too difficult or tedious to use. Theoretically, any food in a given list may be exchanged for any other food in that list, in the amounts recommended. I say "theoretically" because many of the exchangeable foods are not equal in their nutritional or metabolic value. The exchange system operates like a food currency, which allows you a way to measure the types of foods you're eating within each meal and for the day. Each unit of food can be exchanged for another food from that same list. The exchange categories are starch, fruit, milk, vegetables, meat, and fats. For example, a slice of bread has the same value as a small baked potato.

If you are using the exchange system, consider the glycemic value of each food. For example, a slice of bread may be exchanged on the starch list for a potato or another piece of bread. But realize that if the bread is made with soy flour, wheat germ, and bran, it will metabolize more slowly (stabilizing blood sugar) than a piece of white refined-flour bread. The glycemic index can help you determine the best choices for you within the exchange system if you choose to use it.

....

Building Your Medical Team

$\mathcal{W}$ith symptoms like excessive thirst, frequent urination, and possibly rapid weight loss, most people will go to their family doctor. The doctor will generally run through a series of questions to determine whether the patient is manifesting symptoms of diabetes. Then he or she will order a glucose tolerance test to verify the suspicion. This test will reveal the amount of sugar in the bloodstream, which is normally 80 to 110 millimoles per liter (mmol/L). A reading higher than 110 mmol/L would indicate the body is having trouble absorbing sugar. The range of blood glucose control for diabetics needs to be about 120–150. However, blood glucose level goals are set for those with diabetes depending on each person's unique situation. For example, an 80-year-old who lives alone and is newly diagnosed with diabetes may have a goal range between 120 and 200, while a pregnant woman may have a goal of 80–120 before meals and 100–140 one hour after meals. These ranges should be checked quarterly at a doctor's office, as these readings will be more accurate than those given by home glucose meters.

If you have a blood sugar test and your doctor diagnoses anything from a slight case of hypoglycemia to a severe case of diabetes, you will need to begin to build your team of experts to help you get the most up-to-date and effective care possible.

Your Medical Team and You

Begin thinking of yourself as the head of your own medical or health-care team. You are responsible for hiring the team members and coordinating their efforts. As the final decision maker, you need to understand as much as possible about your options in choosing team members, treatment strategies, and the all-important maintenance plan. You need to learn as much as you can about your condition. As you interview medical professionals, remember that you're hiring them and you're paying them to take care of your most valuable asset—your health.

How to Interview Medical Professionals

Part of your job as health-care team leader is to interview the members of the team you are looking to hire. Create your own list of questions or use the list in the "Keeping Records" section in this chapter to aid you in the interviewing process.

Either make copies from this book or take the book with you to appointments. Most health professionals will provide a fifteen-minute interview free of charge if you request it. Call ahead to set up an appointment. Keep in mind that you are hiring them, and you are worth the best care available.

The Team Members

Your health-care team will probably include the following members: an endocrinologist, a nutritionist, a gynecologist (if you're a woman), a dentist or dental hygienist, a naturopathic doctor (N.D.), and possibly an oriental medicine doctor (O.M.D.).

Endocrinologist

Endocrinologists specialize in diseases of the endocrine system and are specially trained to treat diabetes. The pancreas, an endocrine gland, is the key malfunctioning organ in diabetes.

Nutritionist

An appointment with a nutritionist is the first step in taking control of hypoglycemia. Often hypoglycemia can be treated simply with a meal plan, and no further problems occur. At the first sign of blood sugar imbalance, find a whole-foods nutritionist to help you design an individual food plan. The nutritionist can assess your individual micronutrient needs. Nutritionists are trained to interpret lab tests and identify physical signs of nutrient deficiency. They are generally the health professionals with the most focus on nutrient absorption and metabolism. They will help you find the best supplements to meet your needs. These specialists are trained to help you design a meal plan to fill your nutrient and caloric needs, a task that can get fairly complicated when planning around insulin injections.

Registered dietitians (R.D.s) are trained in the use of the American Diabetic Association's food exchange system. They can help you calculate your daily goals for macronutrients (carbohydrates, fats, and proteins) and discuss your needs for vitamins and minerals.

A nutritionist with M.S. after his or her name has a master of science degree; C.N. means certified nutritionist.

Gynecologist

All women past the age of twelve should have a gynecologist on their team. Gynecologists are experts in the female reproductive system. Your family doctor may also serve as your gynecologist.

Dentist or Dental Hygienist

Your family dentist should be informed that you have diabetes.

Naturopathic Doctor

An N.D. is a doctor who is trained in natural health care. N.D.s may use homeopathic medicines, herbs, hydrotherapy, and/or diet therapy as part of their treatments. They treat underlying symptoms to help the patient reach a natural balance by removing the obstacles to health. For example, if a patient has a skin rash, rather than just treating the symptom with cortisone cream, a naturopathic doctor would seek out the reason for the rash (perhaps a food allergy) and treat that underlying condition. An N.D. is an important part of your medical team, because side effects such as candida and food allergies are common problems for people with diabetes. To find an N.D. near you, call the American Association of Naturopathic Physicians at (206) 298-0126.

Oriental Medicine Doctor

O.M.D.s provide acupuncture, herbal treatments, and meal planning advice. Like N.D.s, they treat the underlying conditions of a disease rather than the symptoms.

Developing an Options List

Getting opinions and knowing your options is the first step in interviewing specialists. Here are just a few ways to start your search:

- Referral from your family doctor
- Referral from others with the same condition
- Referral from friends
- Referral from your local pharmacist
- Natural health centers such as Bastyr University in Seattle, Washington, at (206) 523-9585
- On-line services
- Newspapers, magazines, and local phone books

Keeping Records

Keep copies of your medical records and lab results. You'll want to take them to your visits with each of your team members. You may also need copies down the road in case you change team members. File your records in banker's boxes and/or scan them onto a computer disk for storage.

When interviewing practitioners, consider asking these questions:

- What services do you offer?
- What special skills, approach, and types of treatment do you offer?
- How long have you been in practice? (New professionals have the advantage of being fresh out of school, with all the up-to-date research; old-timers have the advantage of years of experience.)

- What degrees or professional training do you have? (This is often revealing about the person's level of expertise, focus, and specialization within a field.)
- What professional associations do you belong to? (Professional organizations are the conduit where specialists get their continuing educations. This is especially important for doctors who have been in practice for more than a few years, as it is easy to get out of date in the quickly changing medical profession.)
- How much time can I expect at each visit? Will you be able to take the time to answer my questions?
- What is the average cost of the initial visit?
- What is the cost for follow-up visits?
- What will be the cost of services, including lab work?
- Are my recent lab tests still valid? (If you are getting a second opinion or recently had lab work done for another doctor, you may want to avoid having to repeat the process.)
- Are you a certified diabetes educator?

Getting the Most Out of Your Office Visit

Be prepared for appointments. If you are organized, you will get more out of your visits and have more time to get your questions answered.

Before Your visit

Think of the questions you have about your condition and what the practitioner should be able to answer for you. Write down your questions. Try to keep them as brief as possible. If you think you will need more than the usual fifteen- to twenty-minute appointment with your practitioner, ask to schedule a longer visit. Plan to take your meal plan and medication records with you.

During the Visit

Take along all of your medications and vitamins in their original bottles. Just scoop them all into a bag and take them along.

This allows your practitioner to see the types and dosages of medications you are taking.

Briefly explain to your doctor the reason for your visit. Stay focused. Explain your problems and symptoms. Answer questions accurately and completely. Be thorough about the medications, vitamins, herbs, alcohol, and tobacco you are using. Let the practitioner know who the members of your medical team are.

Listen carefully. Ask questions if you do not fully understand what your practitioner is recommending and why. Be sure you understand any directions, prescriptions, or exercises. Write down everything important; don't rely on your memory.

Be sure you understand and fully accept the instructions and/or prescriptions before you leave the office so that you are comfortable following them at home. Studies show only one-third of all patients follow their doctor's instructions and more than half fail to take their medications as advised. Tell your doctor if you disagree with or don't think you will follow the recommendations. Let your doctor know before you stop medications or alter dosages.

Leaving a Visit

Before you leave a medical professional's office, you should be able to:

- Describe your condition.
- Define the next appointments and tests and why they are needed.
- Explain your treatment, including medications, therapies, and new protocols.
- State whether and when you need to return to that practitioner.

If you are unclear about any of these, schedule another visit or make an appointment for a phone consultation to get the rest of your questions answered.

Part III

Special Topics

I I

Causes and Triggers
of Diabetes

*T*here are many theories about the causes of diabetes. It is generally believed that there is a genetic code for diabetes that is passed down from our parents, who inherited it from their parents. The code lies dormant in our cells until something triggers its expression. You may have been exposed to several triggers or none of them.

These are just a few of the theories being considered today:

- A family history of diabetes: if someone in your family had diabetes, other family members are more likely to develop diabetes.
- Race or ethnic background: the risk of diabetes is increased in African-American, Hispanic, and some Native American people.
- Viral triggers: the flu, chicken pox, and measles are being considered as catalysts.
- Autoimmune disease: your body's defense system attacks certain healthy cells in your pancreas that produce insulin (beta cells).
- Overweight: the risk increases by 4.5 percent for every 2.2 pounds you gain over your ideal body weight.
- Age: your chance of developing diabetes increases with age.
- Certain drugs: use of blood pressure medications (Thiazide, for example) and steroid medications, such as Prednisone or Decadron, may increase risk.

- Alcohol: your chance of developing diabetes may increase with years of heavy alcohol use.
- Pregnancy: because of the extra demand on a pregnant woman's body, some develop gestational diabetes. For many of these women, blood sugar levels return to normal after childbirth, but their risk of developing diabetes in the future is increased.

Types of Diabetes

Type 1 diabetes mellitus. Genes have been identified that indicate diabetes is a hereditary disease. One in three Americans is believed to carry the genetic predisposition for its development or manifestation. Many people who carry the gene may pass it on to their children without developing the disease themselves. The manifestation of type 1 diabetes is thought to be triggered by a virus or an immune overload of environmental toxins. There is a correlation between babies being fed cow's milk and the development of diabetes later in life. Type 1 diabetes is most common in people under the age of forty who are overweight. They do not produce insulin, so they cannot use sugar as energy, and their blood sugar rises.

Type 2 diabetes mellitus. Type 2 usually develops in people over forty years of age; 90 percent of all people with diabetes are in this category. In type 2 diabetes, the pancreas produces some insulin, but it is not sufficient for normal energy production or it cannot be used effectively. Often the symptoms for diabetes (types 1 and 2) are so obscure that people don't suspect they have diabetes until they have a routine medical examination.

There are, however, warning signs. If you or a family member should have any of the symptoms listed in the following table, you should consult your doctor immediately:

Possible Warning Signs

Type 1	Type 2
Constant urination	Constant urination
Extreme thirst	Extreme thirst
Obvious weakness and fatigue	Itching, dry skin
Irritability	Family history of diabetes
Unusual hunger	Blurred vision
Rapid loss of weight	Excessive weight
	Unexplained weight loss
	Cramps in legs, feet, and fingers
	Slow healing of cuts
	Infections of skin, gums, vagina, or bladder
	Tingling numbness in feet or hands
	Drowsiness or easy fatigue

Moreover, 90 percent of those with type 2 diabetes are overweight at the time of diagnosis. Weight loss, proper meal planning, and regular physical activity are key factors in managing type 2 diabetes mellitus. People who do not eat well and do not exercise properly may need to take an oral glucose-lowering pill or insulin injections. Culture, age, lifestyle, continuously raised blood sugar levels, and stress are all contributing factors. Low birth weight and malnutrition in the womb are also correlated with type 2 development. Unfortunately, in the wealthiest nation in the world, a considerable number of infants are malnourished.

Type 2A obese diabetes. These patients are more than 20 percent over their ideal body weight and have deficiencies in insulin binding sites on target cells stemming from their obesity.

They do not require insulin. Proper meal plans for weight
reduction and maintenance can often reverse the conditions.

Type 2B nonobese diabetes. This subtype of diabetes occurs in people who are not overweight. About 10 percent of those with
type 2 diabetes belong to this group. They do not require
insulin. They frequently have a slowed insulin response to
meals. Numerous small daily meals and proper nutrition make
a tremendous difference for these individuals.

Gestational diabetes. Gestational diabetes develops during pregnancy. Women who develop it are reevaluated after pregnancy, when blood glucose usually returns to normal.
However, 30 to 40 percent of these women will develop diabetes within five to ten years. It is important for them to follow the diabetic eating plan to reduce their risk of developing
the disease later in life.

Secondary diabetes. Secondary diabetes is associated with certain
conditions or syndromes (a pattern of symptoms occurring
together), such as diabetes induced by drugs or chemicals or
by pancreatic or endocrine disease. The endocrine system is
made up of the pancreas and the thyroid, adrenal, pituitary,
and gonad glands. These glands release chemical substances
into the body that regulate and control its various functions.

Possible Triggers

Many factors are being studied to see if and how they increase
the risk of developing diabetes. Among them are the standard
American diet, cow's milk, environmental factors (such as toxins and stress), viruses, autoimmune diseases, and syndrome X
(discussed later in this chapter).

The SAD Connection

SAD stands for the standard American diet, which features a lot
of refined carbohydrates and synthetic sweeteners and not much
fiber. Such eating habits are implicated in the onset of diabetes.

A recent study in the *Journal of the American Medical Association*
revealed that a diet high in fiber and low in sugar may be a major

factor in preventing diabetes. Jorge Salmeron, M.D., and colleagues from the Harvard School of Public Health evaluated data on more than 65,000 American women between the ages of forty and sixty-five. The findings suggest that people can cut their risk of adult-onset diabetes by more than half by replacing junk foods with high-fiber foods like beans, peas, lentils, and whole grains.

Cow's Milk

Ingestion of cow's milk may result in antibodies to, and the destruction of, beta cells in genetically susceptible people. (Karjalainen et al. 1992) Scientists believe that young children have highly permeable intestines for absorbing mother's milk. When they are fed cow's milk, large proteins are transferred into the bloodstream through the gut lining, causing the immune system to respond by producing **antigens** across the gut walls as protection. Our immune system responds to antigens by producing antibodies or immunoglobins by our lymphocytes. There are many different types of immunoglobins such as IgA, IgD, IgE, IgG, and IgM.

Many studies offer significant evidence that exposure to cow's milk at an early age is linked to the development of type 1 diabetes. A study comparing a group of 142 Finnish children with newly diagnosed type 1 to a group of 79 healthy children and 300 adult blood donors found elevated Immunoglobulin G (IgG) antibodies to bovine serum albumin (BSA) in all diabetic patients. (Karjalainen et al. 1992) The Childhood Diabetes in Finland Study Group discovered the siblings of the diabetic children studied who tested positive for islet-cell antibodies had elevated cow's milk proteins. (Vahasalo et al. 1996)

A ten-year study of two thousand newborns in Canada and Finland is now in progress. Researchers are monitoring the development of diabetes in babies given cow's milk during their first nine months.

A French study found a correlation between IgG anti-BSA antibodies and type 1 diabetes. Diabetic patients were found to have elevated anti-bsa levels in 74.4 percent of cases, compared with 5.5 percent of controls. (Levy-Marchal et al. 1995)

Another study found a connection between -casein and type 1 diabetes. It found specific proliferation of T lymphocytes with bovine -casein in 51 percent (24 of 47) of patients with diabetes, compared to 2.7 percent (1 of 36) of healthy subjects. (Cavallo et al. 1996) Of children newly diagnosed with type 1, 55 percent (22 of 40) had enhanced immune response to -lactoglobulin, compared with 22 percent (7 of 32) of healthy children. (Vaarala et al. 1996)

Type 1 diabetes is up to 50 percent higher among children who are bottle-fed. Researchers have discovered that an immune response to the protein can develop in genetically predisposed children. The highest incidence of type 1 diabetes is in Finland, which also has the highest milk consumption in the world. The people of Western Samoa had no known cases of type 1 until they immigrated to New Zealand and drank cow's milk for the first time.

Statistically significant correlations between type 1 and antibodies to cow's milk proteins, particularly bovine serum albumin, have been found. (Karjalainen et al. 1992, Saukkonen et al. 1995 and 1996, Vahasalo et al. 1996) These studies strongly indicate that infants under six months should not be given cow's milk as a substitute for mother's milk. It appears to be a causative factor in the development of juvenile diabetes.

Environmental Factors

Environmental factors encompass toxins as well as both physical and psychological stress. Many toxins have been considered potential triggers at some time. For example:

- food additives
- rat poison
- highly refined foods
- ultraviolet radiation from the sun
- smoked foods
- cassava

Stress is a known trigger for a host of disease states. Cell-damaging stress may weaken the immune system to the point of facilitating diabetes. Many specialists see the growth spurts during childhood, preadolescence, and puberty as a stimulus for diabetes in those with a genetic predisposition.

Noninsulin-requiring diabetes may also be unmasked by physical or emotional stress, such as a serious illness, the death of a spouse, divorce, or the loss of a job. It is not uncommon for a person in the middle years to be admitted to the hospital for a heart attack, stroke, or some other stress-related condition, only to learn that he or she also has diabetes.

Pancreatic Cancer

The islets of Langerhans in the pancreas contain specialized beta cells. These cells produce the hormone insulin, which enters the bloodstream and escorts glucose into cells, which use it for energy. When the beta cells are damaged, they can no longer produce insulin, and diabetes results.

Viruses

The viruses thought to be diabetes triggers include the following:

- mumps (which can cause acute pancreatitis and sometimes hyperglycemia)
- rubella (German measles)
- cytomegalovirus
- herpes
- polio
- tick-borne encephalitis
- ringworm (40 percent of babies with ringworm develop diabetes)
- infectious hepatitis
- coxsackie B

Exposure to an allergen or a virus can trick your immune system into responding with an attack of white blood cells known as T lymphocytes and macrophages. A localized release of cytokines and cytotoxic amounts of nitric oxide and reactive oxygen intermediates contributes to free-radical damage to the pancreas.

This immune response takes place on the surface of the insulin-producing beta cells, which become so damaged that the immune system no longer recognizes them. The immune system then responds as if the beta cells were foreign invaders and attacks them. This destruction is thought to occur over several years. (Foster 1987, Gale 1996)

Some viruses seem to attack the beta cells directly rather than causing an autoimmune reaction. In one study, mumps infection was reported just before the onset of diabetes in 42.5 percent of subjects with type 1, versus a 12.5 percent incidence in the nondiabetic group. (Mijac et al. 1995) Elevated levels of coxsackie B virus IgM antibodies have been reported in patients with newly diagnosed type 1 diabetes. (Schmerthaner 1995)

Screening for Type 1 Diabetes

Only 10 percent of diabetes cases are familial, so it's important to screen the entire population. Evaluations involve both immunological and genetic screening. Markers associated with future-onset diabetes include islet-cell antibodies (ICA) and antibodies against glutamic acid decarboxylase (GAD) and protein tyrosine phosphatase. They are detectable in the blood circulation for years before insulin-dependent diabetes develops. (Gale 1996)

Immune Suppressive Therapy

Now that blood tests are available that reveal whether we have the genes for diabetes or not, we can attempt to prevent the disease. Getting tested for the beta-cell antibodies may be the best defense against developing diabetes.

Immunosuppressive medications are now being investigated as possible intervention therapy. Intensive intravenous insulin therapy is used as an immunization. But vaccinations are not available against potential viral triggers.

Syndrome X

Syndrome X is a set of cardiovascular risk factors that includes a tendency to store fat in the abdominal region, impaired glucose tolerance, high triglycerides, low HDL cholesterol, high blood pressure, high levels of uric acid, and increased apo-B (a component of lipoproteins). The common metabolic factor in cases of syndrome X is elevated insulin levels, which lead to type 2 diabetes.

Syndrome X is often called the insulin resistance syndrome. It is sometimes known as metabolic cardiovascular risk syndrome, atherothrombogenic syndrome, or Reaven's syndrome. Physicians are just beginning to recognize the symptoms of this silent, frequently untreated, but often lethal condition. It's estimated that as much as 25 percent of the cardiovascular disease in men and 60 percent of that in women is the result of syndrome X.

Factors that contribute to its manifestation include a high intake of refined carbohydrates, salt, saturated fat, preservatives, and food colorings. Smoking and a sedentary lifestyle are also common.

Symptoms include those typical of heart disease: shortness of breath; faintness or dizziness; excessive sweating; leg cramps while walking; pain in the shoulders, jaw, and left arm; and chest pain or pressure.

Cardiovascular (heart) disease is a general term associated with hardening of the arteries that supply oxygen to the heart (coronary arteries), reduced blood flow to the heart, high blood pressure, and decreased blood flow to arms and legs (peripheral vascular disease). Heart disease is a leading cause of death for people with diabetes. Men with diabetes have a five times higher rate of developing heart disease than men without it. For women, this rate is even higher. People with diabetes also have an increased chance of developing high blood pressure, which can affect their heart, kidneys, and eyes. Talk to your doctor if your blood pressure is above 130 over 85.

In many ways your heart is a machine, and all machines

require fuel to perform their work. The cells that run your heart pump require fuel that is not only plentiful but also available in a timely fashion. In syndrome X, the levels of your body's fuel (glucose) become unregulated and contribute to the development of heart disease. Let's look at how syndrome X causes fuel production to go wrong. Then we will discuss the carbohydrates that provide glucose and the nutrients that can be used to facilitate and regulate their use in fuel production.

Obesity

It is not the amount of fat a person carries that is related to syndrome X; it is the pattern in which the fat is stored. Men usually store their fat deep in the abdomen (the so-called apple or android shape), while women usually store their fat in their hips, thighs, and upper arms (the so-called pear or gynecoid shape). One out of every four men over the age of forty has excess abdominal fat and insulin resistance. Women are at greater risk of accumulating visceral fat after menopause.

"Apples" are at greater risk for heart disease and insulin resistance than "pears." You do not have to be overweight to have this pattern. To test if you are an apple or a pear, measure the circumference of your waist at the navel and divide it by the largest circumference of your hip. A waist-to-hip ratio greater than 0.9 in men and 0.8 in women is defined as an apple shape.

Abdominal obesity does not specifically cause high cholesterol levels. But it is associated with an increase in an apoprotein called apo-B, which is associated with ischemic heart disease and is present in people with insulin resistance syndrome.

Obesity also decreases the number of receptors on cells so that the normal insulin levels are less than are needed to do the job. Even a moderate weight loss of 10 percent can increase the number of receptors to normal levels. It can also reduce risk factors for type 2, as well as high blood pressure and heart disease, by 20 to 75 percent.

Some 90 percent of those with type 2 diabetes are over-weight. Body fat creates insulin resistance and contributes to the development of insulin-dependent diabetes. Type 2 diabetes has been strongly linked to a high fat intake.

Insulin Resistance

Insulin is the hormone responsible for regulating energy metab-olism. It is produced in the beta cells of the pancreas. Cells in the liver, muscle tissue, and adipose (fat) tissue are most respon-sive to insulin.

When the glucose levels in the blood begin to rise after a meal, insulin is released into the bloodstream to circulate with the glucose molecules. When the two reach a hungry cell, the insulin interacts with the cell, opening the receptors as a key might open a door. This allows not only glucose and insulin but also free fatty acids to enter the cell. Glucose that enters mus-cle tissue is immediately burned for energy if the muscle is exer-cising. If the muscle tissue is at rest the glucose is stored as glycogen, a temporary storage molecule that provides energy between meals. Glucose that enters the liver is also stored as glycogen. After the glycogen storage capacity of the liver cells is filled, any additional glucose absorbed is changed into fatty acids and stored as fat. Glucose that enters fat cells is used to make the glycerol hangers for triglycerides.

Without insulin to open the doors, a cell could be swimming in glucose yet starve to death. This condition of no insulin and high blood sugar (hyperglycemia) is called type 1 diabetes. It results from the destruction of the insulin-producing beta cells of the pancreas.

When insulin is plentiful but unable to unlock enough doors, the cell is said to be insulin resistant. Sometimes this is due to a decrease in the number of receptor-doors or to a defect in some of the locks. This causes insulin blood levels to rise. The body then detects the free glucose molecules and secretes still more insulin. This results in *hyperinsulinemia*, or high blood levels of insulin. The increased levels of insulin are often enough to force glucose into cells so that glucose levels fall to normal as long as insulin levels remain high. Eventually hyperinsulinemia causes the cells to reduce their number of receptor-doors, making the problem worse.

When insulin levels in the blood rise even slightly, the amount of sodium excreted in the urine decreases. This causes sodium retention, which promotes high blood pressure. High insulin levels are also highly toxic to the endothelial cell wall and can cause cell injury that could initiate formation of plaques in the arteries. In the lining of the **arterioles**, insulin stimulates the growth of smooth muscle cells and promotes the formation of cholesterol, triglyceride, and collagen deposits.

Hyperinsulinemia can also cause LDL cholesterol to mutate into a more dangerous form and increases the manufacture of dense, atherogenic LDL in the liver. Insulin resistance is also associated with microvascular angina, chest pain caused by spasms in the coronary arteries.

Finally, insulin resistance increases the reabsorption of sodium from the kidney tubules. This results in an increase in blood volume, causing high blood pressure, which further accelerates the development of cardiovascular disease.

Insulin resistance is a symptom of adult-onset diabetes (also called noninsulin-dependent diabetes mellitus, or NIDDM). Results from the recent multicenter Insulin Resistance and Atherosclerosis Study (IRAS) identified insulin resistance as an independent risk factor for atherosclerosis.

Impaired Glucose Tolerance

As we have seen, when glucose levels in the blood rise, the body responds by releasing insulin. Sometimes, however, the body does not secrete enough insulin to return glucose levels to normal. This results in *hyperglycemia*. When glucose levels are higher than normal but less than in diabetes, impaired glucose tolerance (IGT) occurs. IGT may also be referred to as glucose resistance, decreased glucose tolerance, or glucose intolerance. No matter what the name, the result is the same: not enough insulin is secreted by the pancreas to open the receptor-doors. The body is in effect "insensitive" or "intolerant" to glucose levels.

IGT can be the result of a decrease in the number of beta cells as the result of increased age or faulty genes. It can also be the result of insulin resistance. Stress on the beta cells to secrete the large amounts of insulin needed to overcome insulin resistance can decrease insulin production. The more insulin resistant a person is, the higher his or her plasma glucose. In this instance, serum insulin levels fall while glucose levels remain high.

In people with continual hyperglycemia, the glucose molecule attaches itself to protein molecules, causing protein-to-protein links. In the cardiovascular system, the collagen in the arterial wall can cross-link with the protein portion of LDL particles, binding them so that the LDL particles cannot leave. This contributes to the buildup of LDL cholesterol in the vascular wall.

When protein cross-links with LDL particles in the bloodstream, the LDL structure is altered so that LDL particles are no longer recognized by the receptors responsible for clearing them from circulation. This increases the amount of LDL cholesterol in circulation.

Dietary Sources of Glucose

In the human diet, most of the energy (glucose) that feeds your cells comes from carbohydrates. The type of carbohydrate a glucose molecule comes from has a very strong influence on how this molecule affects the body. Some glucose sources can increase glucose tolerance; others decrease tolerance. Some foods also provide important minerals that affect glucose tolerance.

SIMPLE CARBOHYDRATES

Simple carbohydrate molecules are constructed of one or two monosaccharide sugar rings. The three *monosaccharides* are glucose, fructose, and galactose. These three sugars contain the same number of carbon, hydrogen, and oxygen atoms. Only the arrangement of the atoms is different.

When two of these rings are bonded, they produce the *disaccharides*: sucrose (glucose and fructose); lactose (glucose and galactose); and maltose (glucose and glucose). Sucrose, or white table sugar, is the most common simple sugar. Lactose is the sugar that is found in milk, where it provides energy and enhances the absorption of calcium. Maltose is found only in germinating cereals. The disaccharides are easily broken into monosaccharides in the intestine by their corresponding enzymes: sucrase, lactase, and maltase. The absorbed fructose and galactose are sent to the liver, where their atoms are rearranged into glucose molecules.

Since simple carbohydrates need little digestion, they enter the bloodstream quickly, increasing blood glucose levels and inducing insulin production. This is why you should greatly reduce the amount of sweet foods you eat if you have syndrome X. To slow glucose absorption, never eat sweet foods on an empty stomach. Eating them with protein, fiber, or fat increases the time food spends in the stomach, so glucose enters the blood slowly and insulin levels remain even.

Digestible Complex Carbohydrates

Chains of many simple sugars are complex carbohydrates called *polysaccharides*. The digestible polysaccharides found in food are starch and glycogen. Glucose molecules arranged as linear chains are called amylose and branched chains are called amylopectin. These two starch chains are produced by plants in the form of granules. The size and shape of starch granules differ from plant to plant, giving each type of plant its own unique type of starch with its own blend of amylose and amylopectin.

Starch chains are digested by the body into sugars. Since the end product of starch digestion is glucose, starch can raise insulin and glucose levels in a fashion similar to simple carbohydrates. This rise in insulin and glucose can make the insulin

resistance found in syndrome X much worse. See the last section of this chapter on how to avoid raising insulin levels when
eating complex carbohydrates.

INDIGESTIBLE COMPLEX CARBOHYDRATES

Fiber is composed of cellulose, pectin, algeal substances, gums,
and mucilages. Fiber differs from the other polysaccharides
because it resists digestion by human enzymes and enters the
colon in much the same chemical shape in which it was eaten.
Insoluble fibers, such as cellulose in wheat and rice bran, absorb
and hold water. These fibers increase the bulk of the feces.

Soluble fiber, as the name suggests, dissolves in the watery contents of the colon, giving it a gel-like consistency. Although
resistant to digestion by human enzymes, soluble fiber is readily
digested by the friendly bacteria of the colon. You have probably heard about the ability of soluble fiber to decrease cholesterol
levels. It is thought to do this through two mechanisms.

1. The soluble fiber interacts with the cholesterol-containing
   bile salts released in the duodenum from the liver. They
   bind the cholesterol in the bile so that it cannot be reab-
   sorbed. As a result, the liver must use its own cholesterol
   to replenish the bile salts, and the total amount of cholesterol is decreased.
2. The soluble fibers digested by the colonic bacteria are fermented into gases, lactic acid, and short-chain fatty acids.
   These fermentation products (mostly propionate) are
   absorbed into the bloodstream, where they may influence
   lipid metabolism in the liver.

These fibers also increase the time that other foods in the
same meal spend in the stomach, slowing their absorption rate.
This results in a more constant supply of energy for the cell
and lower glucose and insulin levels in the blood. Increasing
the soluble fiber in your diet is one of the best ways to treat
syndrome X.

Treatments for Syndrome X

The best treatment for syndrome X is good nutrition. Cut way back on saturated fats and cholesterol (meats, dairy products, and eggs) and eat more fiber-rich foods (legumes, grains, vegetables, and fruits). Eliminate (or at least cut back on) coffee and increase your intake of essential fatty acids.

Greatly reduce the amount of sweet (simple carbohydrate) foods you eat. To slow glucose absorption, never eat sweet foods on an empty stomach; always eat them with protein, fiber, or fat. These nutrients increase the time food spends in the stomach so that glucose enters the blood slowly and insulin levels remain even.

To avoid raising insulin levels when eating complex carbohydrates:

- Stress starches that have a high amylose content. A diet rich in amylose starch has been shown to improve insulin tolerance and decrease triglyceride levels.
- Do not overcook pasta and starchy vegetables such as potatoes and yams. Cooking food softens the cells that contain starch, bursting them open and making starch more available to the digestive enzymes of the gastrointestinal tract. The longer a starchy food is cooked, the faster it will elevate glucose and insulin levels.
- Because large pieces of food take longer to digest and absorb, do not mash or puree starchy foods. Serve potatoes in slices rather than mashed. Choose larger sizes of pasta. Avoid vegetable juices on an empty stomach.
- Eat whole, unrefined starchy foods such as brown rice and steel-cut oats. Their fat and fiber will slow digestion and absorption and blunt the insulin response. By contrast, instant white rice and quick rolled oats elevate blood sugar levels too quickly.
- The protein in high-protein wheat, legumes, nuts and seeds, fish, and lean meat will also blunt the insulin

response. Add a little protein to all of the meals you eat, including snacks.

The other component of treatment is regular exercise. Get at least thirty minutes of aerobic (oxygen-using) exercise at least three times a week. And while you're at it, stop smoking. See Chapter 14 for more information on the benefits of exercise.

Treatment for syndrome X may include medication and, in extreme cases, surgery.

12

Emergency Planning

$\mathcal{P}$lanning ahead can help you cope with blood sugar emergencies.

Your Emergency Kit

Always carry an emergency kit with you that contains the following items:

- *Glucose.* Carry several doses of glucose tabs or gel.
- *Insulin.* Have enough insulin and syringes to last several days.
- *Food.* Aseptic packages of soy milk and juice can be kept unrefrigerated for up to a year if unopened. Keep a few in your car, in your purse, and at your office.
- *Water replacement.* A plastic bottle of water will keep indefinitely if unopened.
- *Emergency phone numbers.* Include numbers for your endocrinologist and the hospital.

What Is Hypoglycemia?

*Hypo*glycemia means *low* blood sugar. This condition happens when you have too much insulin and not enough sugar in your body. In the case of diabetes, hypoglycemia can occur from too much insulin or oral glucose-lowering medication. Low blood sugar reaction (extreme hypoglycemia) is also known as insulin reaction.

Causes and Symptoms of Hypoglycemia

Causes of hypoglycemia include missing a meal, being more active than usual, not eating enough, not eating when ill, eating later than usual, taking too much medication, and/or drinking alcohol.

Early symptoms include weakness, shakiness, hunger, dizziness, sweating, trembling, pounding heart, pale skin, and confusion. Late symptoms include headache, irritability, impaired coordination, numbness in mouth, and fainting.

Treating and Preventing Hypoglycemia

In a low blood sugar emergency (readings of less than seventy milligrams per deciliter [mg/dl]), eat sugar or sugar-containing foods. Eat just one item from the following list and wait fifteen minutes, then check your blood sugar. If it's less than eighty milligrams per deciliter, eat another serving. If your next scheduled meal is more than forty-five minutes away, eat some protein-containing food, such as peanut butter and bread or cheese and crackers. This should prevent another low blood sugar reaction. Eat one or two of the following items in a low blood sugar emergency:

- ½ cup orange or apple juice
- 1 tablespoon honey
- 2 or 3 glucose tabs or 1 tube of glucose gel (available at most pharmacies)
- 4 to 6 hard candies (caramels are also effective)
- 1 tablespoon brown sugar
- 1 tablespoon corn syrup

When to Call Your Doctor

- If you have blood sugar readings of less than 70 mg/dl three days in a row
- If you have blood sugar readings of more than 180 three days in a row
- If you have even one blood sugar reading of 300 or more
- If you have moderate to large ketones in your urine

What Is Hyperglycemia?

*Hyper*glycemia is the term for *high* blood sugar. This condition happens when your body has too much sugar and not enough insulin. High blood sugar causes a host of uncomfortable symptoms. When you have it for long periods of time, complications increase considerably. Nerve, eye, and blood vessel damage are common effects of long-term uncontrolled blood sugar.

Causes and Symptoms of Hyperglycemia

Causes of hyperglycemia include skipping or forgetting to take insulin or oral medication, eating high-calorie foods, having an infection and/or illness, experiencing increased stress, and being less active than usual.

Hyperglycemia has a variety of symptoms, including increased thirst, blurred vision, frequent urination, fatigue (weak, tired feeling), sugar in urine, weight loss, increased appetite, blood sugar more than 180 milligrams per deciliter, vaginal and skin infections, and slow healing of cuts and sores.

Treating and Preventing Hyperglycemia

Test your blood sugar frequently. If it's over 240 milligrams per deciliter, test urine for ketones. Call your doctor if your blood sugar before breakfast is more than 180 milligrams per deciliter three days in a row.

Do not consume sugary foods or drinks. Follow your meal plan, exercise program, and medication routine.

Recommended Range for Blood Sugar

Time of Test	Normal
Before breakfast	70–120 mg/dl
1 hour after eating	Less than 180 mg/dl
2 hours after eating	Less than 150 mg/dl
At bedtime	120–140 mg/dl
At 3:00 A.M.	More than 65 mg/dl

What Is Ketoacidosis?

Hyperglycemia can lead to an emergency condition known as *ketoacidosis*. When your cells are not absorbing sugar, they give the signal that they are starving. So the cells begin to metabolize healthy body tissue such as fats and proteins. When fat is metabolized, ketones appear in the blood and urine. Ketones can be dangerous because they create an acidic state in the blood. People who are taking insulin are at greatest risk of developing ketoacidosis.

Causes and Symptoms of Ketoacidosis

The causes of ketoacidosis are the same as those of hyperglycemia. By recognizing and treating early signs of hyperglycemia, you can avoid ketoacidosis.

Symptoms of ketoacidosis include loss of appetite; abdominal pain; nausea and vomiting; reddened, warm skin; headache; deep, rapid breathing; drowsiness; fruity-smelling breath; restlessness; frequent urination; and increased thirst.

If you have any of these symptoms, test your blood sugar level and test your urine for ketones. Call your doctor if your blood sugar is more than 240 milligrams per deciliter or you have ketones in your urine.

Treating and Preventing Ketoacidosis

Treatment may include insulin and fluids as ordered by your doctor. Ketoacidosis is serious and can result in coma or death if untreated.

To prevent ketoacidosis, stick to your medication, mealtimes and food quantities, exercise, and blood sugar testing plan.

Sick Days

Illness can throw off even the most carefully planned regimen. Flu, fever, cold, vomiting, diarrhea, and infection all take their toll. But even when you are ill and vomiting, it is important to take your insulin or oral medication. You may be able to tolerate liquid foods such as vegetable or fruit juices.

When you are ill or have an infection:

- Check blood sugar every four hours.
- Check urine for sugar and ketones every four hours.
- Check temperature.
- Drink liquids as often as possible.
- Sip one tablespoon of liquid every fifteen minutes or one-half cup every hour.

Call the doctor if your blood sugar readings are higher than 240 milligrams per deciliter or lower than 70 milligrams per deciliter or if there are ketones in your urine. Also call if you cannot keep liquids or solids down or if you have a fever or diarrhea or are vomiting.

Here are some foods to eat when you're sick. Also, try adding vitamin supplements such as flaxseed oil, powdered vitamin C, protein powder, and herbs to smoothies or shakes.

- plain yogurt
- oatmeal
- fresh vegetable juices
- V-8 or other canned vegetable juices
- vegetable broth or bouillon

13

Oral Medications, Insulin, and Nutrient Interactions

*A*ll medications add an element of complexity and risk to your health. By controlling your blood sugar primarily through diet and exercise, you can reduce your dependence on medications—and in some cases eliminate them.

Oral Medications

Oral glucose-lowering medication is available for people with type 2 diabetes, prescribed to be taken alone or with insulin. Medications of every type cause complex chemical reactions. These reactions may hinder absorption of specific nutrients or cause a higher uptake of others.

Oral medication can help control blood sugar only in combination with a proper diet, exercise, and regular blood sugar testing. When your medications are prescribed, you should also be given instructions, which should include the time of day to take them, side effects to watch for, and your doctor or pharmacist's phone number to call if you experience unusual side effects.

How Oral Agents Work

Oral medications slow down the digestion of carbohydrates by delaying absorption from the small intestine into the bloodstream, thus reducing the peaks of blood sugar. Some increase glucose uptake by the muscles, decrease glucose output of the liver, and/or increase insulin output of the pancreas. Generally, these oral hypoglycemic medications slow down absorption, so they may cause abdominal pain, gas, and diarrhea. These side effects are usually mild and decrease over time.

Insulin

It is estimated that insulin-dependent diabetes makes up about 3 to 5 percent of all cases. When insulin is absent, the cells are in a state of starvation, while an excess of sugar (in the form of glucose) floats around in the blood unable to reach them. This state of high blood sugar is called hyperglycemia. The body literally begins to starve and feed upon itself, causing extreme weakness. Despite eating vast amounts of food, the person remains in a condition of starvation until adequate insulin is available to get the food to the cells.

Symptoms include:

- weakness
- excessive thirst
- frequent urination
- irritability
- nausea
- hunger
- weight loss
- fasting plasma glucose level of 126 milligrams per deciliter or greater on at least two occasions
- plasma glucose level of 200 milligrams per deciliter or greater at two hours and on at least one other occasion during a two-hour glucose tolerance test

In hyperglycemia, body fat is burned as an alternate fuel, which creates a by-product called ketone bodies as a source of energy. But ketones cause a dangerous accumulation of acids and a state of ketoacidosis. (For more about ketones, see Chapter 12.)

Some medications and supplements may interfere with insulin's activity, so it is best to take them at a different time of day from when you take your insulin. Check with your doctor to make sure any other medications you may be taking will not interfere with the insulin's effectiveness.

Certain vitamin and mineral deficiencies also inhibit insulin's effectiveness. For example, chromium and magnesium are necessary for insulin to do its job. If you have high blood sugar levels that you cannot reduce with your diet, you may be experiencing a reduction in insulin's effectiveness. Nutrient deficiencies should be considered. Your doctor can order blood tests to find out if this is the problem.

If you are diagnosed with type 1 diabetes, your endocrinologist will set up a personalized insulin schedule so that you can adjust your own insulin at home when necessary.

Types of Insulin
Insulin is injected under the fat of the skin. It is usually extracted from the pancreases of cows and pigs or made in a lab through genetic engineering to be similar to human insulin. Insulin contains 100 units of insulin per milliliter, so it is called U100. It comes in formulas that work at four different speeds.

VERY FAST ACTING
Other names: Humalog, Lispro
Action time: starts to act 15 minutes after injection
Peak: 45–90 minutes after injection
Duration of effect: 4 hours

FAST ACTING
Other names: also known as soluble insulin and often called regular insulin
Action time: starts to act 30 minutes after injection
Peak: 2–3 hours after injection
Duration of effect: 8 hours

SLOW ACTING
Other names: Isophane, NPH, or Lente
Action time: starts to act 2–3 hours after injection
Peak: 8–16 hours after injection
Duration of effect: 24 hours
Note: these contain added protein or zinc to extend their activity.

VERY SLOW ACTING
Other names: Ultralente
Action time: starts to act in 4–6 hours
Peak: 8–20 hours
Duration of effect: 24–48 hours (generally 36 hours)

The Food and Insulin Equation

Make food choices that fit your insulin activity. Timing meals and snacks to correlate with your insulin schedule will keep the fuel burning at just the right level. Your insulin should be timed to correspond with your usual intake of food.

The effects of insulin depend on:
- the type of insulin you take
- your food choices
- your meal and snack timing
- how hard you exercise
- how long you exercise
- what time of day you exercise

Insulin is working effectively for you when no sugar is spilling into your urine (urine tests show 0) and your blood tests show between 80 and 140 milligrams of glucose per deciliter.

Insulin reactions can happen when:
- you take too much insulin
- you take too many antidiabetic pills
- you get more exercise than normal, which drops your blood sugar too low
- you do not eat enough food to compensate for the amount of insulin taken
- you do not eat enough food at the right time to compensate for the insulin's peak

If blood sugar drops too low, you will become hypoglycemic. A half cup of fruit juice will usually bring your blood sugar back up to a safe level. If blood sugar is so low that you begin to experience the early signs of insulin shock (confusion, weakness, sweaty palms, nausea), consume a sugary drink or candy immediately. After you have some cola, fruit juice, or candy, do a blood sugar test. If blood sugar readings are still too low, contact your doctor.

Low Blood Sugar Fifteen to Thirty Rule

If you have a low blood sugar reading, take fifteen grams of fast-acting carbohydrate, such as fruit juice or sugar-containing foods. Wait fifteen to thirty minutes and recheck your blood sugar before eating more. Remember that your blood sugar will feel low for a lot longer than it actually is.

Monitoring Your Medications

You are the one most closely tracking your drugs. All medications have some implications, and it is important to know what you are taking and why. If your medications cause malabsorption of nutrients, you may develop nutrient deficiencies. Your pharmacist should be able to tell you if any of your medications block nutrient absorption. If they do, you will need to take them separately from your food and/or vitamin and mineral supplements (which will also be an important part of your program).

Taking notes is a good idea. It is easy, especially when taking multiple medications, to forget why you are taking something and who told you to take it. Keep a worksheet on each of your medications in your medical and health file at home. Note the date that you began taking the drug and when you stop taking it. Keep inserts from medications and read the fine print. Ask your pharmacist about insert information.

Be sure you understand which medications your diabetes specialist has recommended and why. Keep your own records so that you can refer to them if you are ever in doubt. Be sure you know whether your medication will cause absorption problems with food, supplements, or other medications. Here is a sample worksheet that you may want to copy and fill out for each medication you take.

Worksheet for Recording Medication Information

Generic and product name _____

_____

Why am I taking this medication? _____

_____

What short-term side effects and nutritional implications does

this medication have? _____

_____

What long-term side effects and nutritional implications does

this medication have? _____

_____

What lifestyle or meal planning changes will I have to make

while taking this medication? _____

_____

What medications might interact with this one? _____

_____

What vitamins or minerals might I need to supplement

because I am taking this medication? _____

_____

What time of day should I take this medication? _____

_____

Should I have food at the time I take this medication? _____

_____

14

The Importance of Exercise

*R*egular exercise is critical for the proper digestion of food, regulation of blood sugar, transportation of nutrients, and efficient functioning of all of your body's organs.

Health Benefits of Exercise

Getting your body moving has many benefits. Exercise reduces blood sugar by burning it as fuel and minimizes extreme fluctuations. It also helps you take off unwanted pounds, which inhibit the function of insulin receptor sites, and it raises your metabolic rate. Regular workouts decrease dependence on diabetic medications and insulin. They diminish the risk of heart disease by lowering blood pressure and body fat and increase the ability to utilize insulin. Studies show that people who work out have a reduced risk of kidney, heart, foot, and eye complications.

Moving your body every day sends blood sugar into the muscles to be used when needed later on, reduces the chemical effects of stress (which raises blood sugar levels), and sends oxygen and nutrients in the blood to all of your body's tissues. This means more oxygen to the brain, which improves thinking and problem solving.

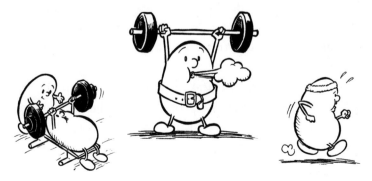

And that's not all. Exercise balances hormones, which improves your mood and sense of well being. It reduces cholesterol and blood lipids and helps reduce damaging homocysteine levels.

Your Exercise Routine

Designing your personal exercise routine starts with choosing a type of exercise that you enjoy. If you are free of diabetic complications, work up slowly to a half hour a day of moderate exercise. If you already have such symptoms as atherosclerosis, retinopathy, or neuropathy, consult your physician or an exercise specialist for types of exercise that are appropriate for you. A trainer can help you choose the type of activity; advise you on the intensity, duration, and frequency; and make the necessary modifications as you progress.

Remember to avoid exercising when your insulin is peaking (usually dinnertime). Avoid exercising within one hour of taking insulin, as this may cause a low blood sugar reaction. The best time to exercise is a half hour to an hour after eating. Drink plenty of water before, during, and after exertion. Be sure to test your blood sugar before and after exercise. If your blood sugar is 120 milligrams per deciliter or lower before you start, eat a snack. If your blood sugar is 300 or higher, wait until it is below 300 to begin exercising.

Exercise with someone who knows you have diabetes and knows what to do if you have a low blood sugar reaction. Wear athletic shoes and a medical ID tag or carry an identification card that states you have diabetes. Stretch for fifteen minutes before you begin, holding each stretch for at least thirty seconds to get lasting benefit.

Modify your insulin or oral medication program and food intake to match your exercise program with the supervision of your doctor. When you are ill, it is best to avoid all but the mildest activities.

When Not to Exercise

WARNING: When your blood sugar level is above 300, exercise could be harmful, because there is not enough insulin available to transport the necessary glucose into the muscles. Exercise will increase ketones and adrenaline will raise blood sugar even higher. Lower your sugar level before you begin.

Here are some easily accessible activities for a regular exercise program:

- brisk walking
- bicycling
- dancing
- in-line skating
- swimming
- tennis
- yoga

Exercise and the Little People

Moving your body helps the little people of the transportation system do their jobs by increasing the movement of the lymph fluids, which contain white blood cells. This enhances the effectiveness of the immune system. Lymph fluid does not have its own motility system: it relies on the movement of the blood through the blood vessels, which lie next to the lymph vessels all over the body. When blood pumps and the blood vessels dilate, they push in on the lymph vessels, which pushes the lymph along. Movement also increases oxygen intake and nutrient distribution.

15

Water Quality

*N*ext to oxygen, water is the most essential element for the survival of human life. Approximately 60 percent of an adult human body is water; brain tissues have an 85 percent water content. Clearly, water plays a critical part in your body's function.

The amount of water you need can be calculated by your body weight.

Body weight (lbs) ÷ 2 = number of ounces per day

Ounces ÷ 8 = number of glasses per day

Example: 120 lbs ÷ 2 = 60 ounces per day

60 ounces ÷ 8 = 7.5 glasses per day

Health Benefits of Water

Water is important for health because it

- carries nutrients and oxygen to the cells,
- aids in digestion and absorption of foods,
- regulates body temperature,
- cushions the joints and protects tissues and organs from shock and injury, and
- removes toxins and wastes from the body.

When your body is lacking in water, all bodily functions are affected. Chronic dehydration may be the cause of a number of disease processes that are currently treated with prescription drugs when simply adding the much-needed water to the diet might help as much. The range of diseases investigated includes asthma, peptic ulcers, allergies, hypertension, and migraine headaches, as well as insulin-dependent diabetes. Scientists even suggest that diabetes may be the end result of a water deficiency in the brain, to the point that its neurotransmitter systems—

particularly the serotonergic system—are affected. A balance between water and salt is needed for neurotransmission mechanisms to function properly, and blood sugar levels rise in circulation in response to a chronic reduction of water and salt in the body.

We need to realize how much our bodies depend on water and make sure we consume a minimum of six to eight 8-ounce glasses a day. If you happen to live in a hot climate, exercise a great deal, are experiencing a fever, or have a kidney disease, you need to increase the amount of water you consume.

Contaminants

Where do we get our eight glasses of water? That question is on the minds of many as the water industry grows by leaps and bounds in response to the problems of contamination that we now face in our limited water supplies. Approximately 70 percent of the Earth's surface is covered with water, but only 1 percent of that is potable (available as a source of drinking water). According to *Consumer Reports*, "No area of the country is free of problems." These problems include volatile organic compounds (VOCs), nitrates, parasitic cysts, lead, endocrine disrupters, trihalomethanes (THMs), asbestos, and radon.

Volatile Organic Compounds

VOCs are a class of organic chemicals that include herbicides, pesticides, and other chemicals that vaporize at low temperatures. They become virtually undetectable in drinking water because they can't be tasted or smelled or seen. They can be toxic and are associated with cancer and damage to the nervous system, brain, liver, and kidneys, as well as potential damage to the immune and reproductive systems.

Nitrates

Nitrates are chemicals generally found in rural areas where agricultural fertilizers are used. They are also associated with higher levels of herbicides and pesticides. The greatest risk is to infants and ill or immunocompromised individuals because the nitrates convert to nitrites via intestinal bacteria, possibly altering the hemoglobin molecule so it cannot carry oxygen.

Parasitic Cysts

Several cysts that enter our water systems made recent head-lines by infecting large communities with choleralike illnesses. A few years ago, cryptosporidium claimed the lives of more than a hundred people in Milwaukee and sickened an additional four hundred thousand. Giardia, also known as "beaver fever" owing to its former association with remote hiking and camping experiences, is now estimated to cause over four thousand hospital admissions and five to ten waterborne outbreaks annually. For healthy individuals, the diarrhea, cramps, nausea, vomiting, headaches, and fever are an uncomfortable inconvenience. For the ever-increasing immunocompromised population, however, these symptoms can be life threatening. Vital organs such as the kidneys, liver, lungs, gallbladder, and pancreas can be severely and permanently damaged. Dialysis patients and people with kidney disease are in the severe risk category.

Lead

Many articles have been written on the effects of the heavy metal lead, which is taken into the body through the air we breathe, the water we drink, and sometimes the plates we eat from. Our single largest source of lead is corroded water pipes, brass faucets, and solder in plumbing installed before 1986, when lead solder was banned by the Environmental Protection Agency (EPA).

Lead has been found to cause a number of health problems, including high blood pressure, cancer, and slowed nerve response. Lead is especially dangerous to infants and children. It causes stunted growth, hearing damage, reduced IQ and retardation, hyperactivity, and a multitude of impairments in such areas as reading, writing, math, memory, language, and concentration. The damage is cumulative and generally believed to be irreversible.

Endocrine Disrupters

Endocrine disrupters are chemicals from industrial waste that are found in our water supply. They can behave like hormones, causing disruption and/or disease in the endocrine, immune, and reproductive systems. The list of potential problems is long, including impaired memory, birth defects, cancer, loss of muscle tone and reflexes, stunted growth, and behavior problems. Reproductive system difficulties include stunted genitals, low sperm counts, endometriosis, infertility, and ectopic pregnancies.

Trihalomethanes

THMs are disinfectant by-products formed when chlorine and other chemicals used to disinfect our water supply combine with organic matter in nature. Some scientists consider them the greatest threat posed in our water systems because they are always present in most areas and are associated with five thousand to eight thousand bladder and rectal cancers per year in the United States.

Asbestos

Asbestos in drinking water generally occurs naturally in the earth, but artificial asbestos has been used as a structural material for concrete pipes used for transporting drinking water. High levels in the drinking water have been associated with colorectal cancer.

Radon

Certain areas of the United States, particularly the Northeast, have radon in groundwater and wells. This radioactive gas is a by-product of uranium, which is found in the Earth's crust.

Radon can be released into the air and breathed through showers, dishwashing, and laundry; it may increase the risk of lung cancer.

Turbidity

Turbidity is the cloudiness present in the water. It can be caused by a number of factors, such as surface water treatment and suspended materials. In and of itself it does not pose a health risk. It does, however, interfere with the process of sterilization and can be associated with THMS.

Who's Most at Risk?

WARNING: With all contaminants, infants, small children, elderly people, and immunocompromised individuals are in the highest risk category.

The Water Options

The drinking-water industry is racing to meet consumers' demands for safe and better-tasting water in response to their concerns about contaminants. There are seemingly countless bottled-water companies with an ever-widening range of flavors and "textures" to choose from. It is important to know that not all bottled waters are the same. To date, bottled water is required to meet only the standards of local tap water. There is also no standard labeling to enable consumers to compare the varieties. Terms like "mineral water" may mean very different things from one state to another. Here are some basic categories:

Distilled water can be obtained from any source and processed by a method of purification called distillation, in which it is evaporated and then condensed.

Drinking water is a loosely used term. It can be water from any source point and any level of sterilization or processing.

Mineral water has a concentration of total dissolved solids (TDS). It can be obtained from any source and the label should specify whether the mineral content is natural or added. The amount of TDS varies greatly from state to state, but there is no standard of quality from any location.

Sparkling water includes club soda, seltzer, and any other waters that contain carbon dioxide, either naturally or added.

Spring water should be just what it says—from a naturally occurring spring. If it is, the word "natural" generally appears on the label. Otherwise, it may have been processed (perhaps by filtration or added carbonation). Spring water can be naturally carbonated and can come from an artesian well (where the groundwater is held between two impermeable layers and its own natural pressure forces it to the surface).

Still water is any water without carbonation or bubbles. This water can come from a spring, a municipal source, or anywhere else. It can be distilled, natural, or processed.

Standards for Drinking Water

Currently, the rules and regulations of the bottled-water industry are no more stringent than those for tap water, which comes under the jurisdiction of the Food and Drug Administration at the federal level. Many companies hold themselves to a high health standard and attempt to observe sterility at each stage of possible contamination. But, unfortunately, not all states require registration or certification of bottle handlers or inspection of plants. There have been many documented cases of contaminants, including bacterial, particulate, and chemical types.

If bottled water doesn't suit your needs, there are alternatives in water treatment technologies (discussed later in this chapter). For comparisons and certification of specific drinking-water systems, NSF (National Sanitation Foundation) International is the internationally recognized, third-party organization that sets the rules to make sure the system meets strict public health standards. For NSF to certify a water treatment system, it must meet five conditions:

1. All contaminant-reduction claims must be accurate.
2. The system must not add anything harmful to the water.
3. The system must be structurally sound.
4. Advertising, literature, and labeling must not be misleading.
5. The materials and manufacturing must not change (or the product must be recertified).

NSF conducts inspections to ensure that any given company continues to meet the requirements.

Two additional organizations are responsible for aspects of our drinking-water standards: the EPA and the Water Quality Association (WQA). The EPA sets these standards and monitors public water utilities. It determines and sets limits on which contaminants are important relative to health and public safety. Since the EPA has complete authority over drinking water from public water supplies, it is authorized to step in to enforce the standards when states fail to do so. It sets the standards for maximum contaminant levels "at a level at which, in the administrator's judgment based on such report, no known or anticipated adverse effects on the health of persons occur and which allows an adequate margin of safety." Unfortunately, the EPA has set maximum contaminant levels for only a hundred or so of the possible thirty thousand hazardous substances found in tap water.

Regarding home water treatment technology, the EPA defers to NSF or the WQA, an international trade association that represents the water treatment industry (specific firms and individuals that design, manufacture, and sell products for water quality). The WQA tests and certifies for industry standards such as chlorine reduction, taste and odor, and particulate-matter reduction. Because it is not a third-party source, the WQA's certification is not considered objective.

For information, contact:

NSF International
3475 Plymouth Rd., P.O. Box 1468
Ann Arbor, MI 48106
http://www.nsf.org
www.nsf.org

EPA Office of Drinking Water (WH-550A)
401 M St., SW
Washington, D.C. 20460
http://www.epa.gov
www.epa.gov

WQA Consumer Affairs Department
P.O. Box 606
Lisle, IL 60532
http://www.wqa.org
www.wqa.org

Water Purification Systems

Home water purification systems generally use one or more of three basic types of water purification: distillation, reverse osmosis, and activated carbon. Each method removes different contaminants and operates differently, so it is important to examine the systems and compare laboratory testing to determine which one will suit your needs. Ask these basic questions before purchasing your water treatment system: Does NSF International certify the system? What is it certified for? (Numbers indicate specific standards as categorized by NSF.)

Contaminant Removal Comparison of Water Purification Systems

Aesthetic Effects

Contaminant	Granular Activated Carbon	Activated Carbon Block	Distillation	Reverse Osmosis
Chlorine	yes	yes	some	no
Particulate matter	most	yes	yes	yes

Health Effects

Contaminant	Granular Activated Carbon	Activated Carbon Block	Distillation	Reverse Osmosis
Asbestos	some	yes	yes	yes
Cysts	some	yes	some	some
Heavy metals	no	yes	yes	yes
Minerals	no	no	yes	yes
Pesticides	some	yes	some	no
Turbidity	most	yes	most	yes
THMS	some	yes	some	some
VOCS	no	yes	some	some

There are more than twenty-five hundred water treatment devices on the market. Here's an overview of the technologies involved.

Distillation uses electricity to heat water to boiling, creating vapor that then cools and returns to liquid. Distillation is effective for killing cysts and reducing heavy metals. The drawbacks are in the use of electricity, the removal of potentially beneficial minerals, and the fact that the volatile chemicals can be recondensed into a liquid state, back into the water source.

Reverse osmosis uses a semipermeable membrane and pressure to force water to leave behind suspended contaminants and pass through to a holding tank. Like distillation, reverse osmosis is a slow process. Three or four gallons of water are shunted or lost for every gallon of drinking water produced. This technology removes heavy metals and minerals but is not as effective in removing the vocs and thms (pesticides). Both distillation and reverse osmosis systems are often paired with granular activated carbon to aid in the removal of chlorine and chemicals.

Granular activated carbon is the type of filter that fits on the end of the faucet. It is designed primarily for aesthetic water treatment, removing enough chlorine to change the taste and odor of the water and not much else. Since the water is flowing through a bed of relatively loose charcoal granules, it may channel around these granules and contaminants will not be adsorbed. It is important to change the filters often because if the charcoal is not treated with silver nitrate, the loose carbon bed may become a breeding ground for bacteria.

Pitchers/Carafes are filters, often of granular carbon or mixed-media material. They're also designed to improve taste and odor. Some remove lead as well as chlorine, but they don't remove the other contaminants that are of health concern. They can filter only a limited amount of water at any given time, so they are best used on demand or to store water in the refrigerator. These filters require frequent changes, so the expense may escalate well beyond the initial investment.

Solid carbon block is perhaps the easiest, most effective technology available for home use. This system employs a three-stage filtering process: a cellulose prefilter; a compressed, solid carbon block; and an insoluble polyethylene filter that strains smaller than a micron. It combines the technology of mechanical straining (to remove solid and semisolid contaminants that can cause premature clogging) and electrokinetic adsorption (to reduce colloidal contaminants down to the submicron range).

The largest manufacturer of solid carbon block systems has recently created an improved filter. Models that sit on the countertop are available as well as ones that easily install under the sink and deliver purified water from a separate spigot. They come in a range of filtration capacities and have the most effective ratings from NSF for the removal of all contaminants tested.

The following water treatments are less commonly used in home applications:

Mixed-media (KDF, ATS) filters are designed to reduce a specific contaminant. They are very efficient relative to that contaminant. KDF filters are specific to chlorine reduction, while ATS filters are designed for lead removal. Their performance for additional contaminants varies.

Ozonation and ultraviolet are more commonly utilized in public water treatment than in home systems. Ozonation uses oxygen to superoxygenate water and kill bacteria. It takes a long contact time with the water to be effective. Ultraviolet radiation is used for bacterial reduction in some applications. It requires the water to be relatively free of turbidity, since the light must penetrate every portion of the water to eliminate each bacterium.

Ion exchange or water softeners are used to alter water hardness. They generally work by exchanging sodium for calcium or magnesium ions in a bed of resin. They are neither purifiers nor filters.

Special Circumstances

If you receive your water from a common city (municipal) source, your needs may differ from those of your friends in the country who drink from a well. City water is generally chlorinated because this is the least expensive way for large water treatment facilities to eliminate the greatest amount of bacteria at any given time.

Wells are less likely to be treated in any manner but should always be tested for possible contamination for your health and safety. Some wells do have a chlorination system for bacterial reduction, or a water softener may be added if the water is hard and full of minerals. A high level of sulfur can be problematic due to the odor, while iron in the water may taste like blood. These problems may require even more refined treatment or a combination of treatments.

The newest class of solid carbon block filtration systems offers special replacement filters to address certain mineral issues, but it is important to know your water source. Is it a shallow well? An artesian well? Is it near a stream or other body of water? Near a golf course? An agricultural area? Check with a professional about well contaminants.

There are many possible avenues of contamination of drinking water, including the chlorine used to disinfect your water as it comes into your home. Purifying your water at home is the safest and most economical method to ensure removal of chemicals found in municipal and well water. Solid carbon block filtration has received the highest ratings in all categories tested by NSF International for municipal water. If you have well water, know its source and have it tested by a lab to determine which system or combination of systems will take care of your special needs. Drinking at least eight glasses of pure water each day is a key component of good health.

16

Reading Food Labels

$\mathcal{M}$ost foods now carry labels detailing nutrition facts. The labels make it easier to choose healthy foods and control diabetes. Reading labels reveals information that will help you determine if foods fit into your meal plan. It's a good idea to make this a regular part of your shopping experience.

Interpreting Nutrition Facts

The Nutrition Facts food labeling is now used uniformly in accordance with the Food and Drug Administration's new federal food labeling regulations. All food packages are required to provide certain information so you can learn more about the foods you are buying.

These labels reveal carbohydrate, protein, fat, sodium, cholesterol, fiber, and generally a few selected vitamins and minerals, listed as a percentage of daily value. The column headed "% Daily Value" shows how the food fits into a reference meal plan of 2,000 calories and 65 grams of fat per day. Ingredients are listed in descending order of predominance by weight. So the first ingredient listed is the one there is the most of and the last is the one there is the least of.

Similar food products now have standard serving sizes, which makes it easier to compare foods. The new food labels list calories per serving, total fat, saturated fat, cholesterol, sodium, total carbohydrate, dietary fiber, sugars, and protein content. All components are given in grams or milligrams per serving and as percentages of daily value. This information will make it easier to purchase foods that fit into your meal plan and help control your blood sugar, cholesterol, blood pressure, and weight.

Here's a breakdown of the items on a typical food label.

Nutrition Facts
Serving Size 1/2 cup (123g)
Servings Per Container approx. 3.5˙

Amount Per Serving		
Calories 60	Calories from Fat 0	
		% Daily Value˙
Total Fat 0g		**0%**
Saturated Fat 0g		**0%**
Cholesterol 0mg		**0%**
Sodium 10mg		**0%**
Potassium 80mg		**2%**
Total Carbohydrate 13g		**4%**
Dietary Fiber 1g		**4%**
Sugars 12g		
Protein 0g		

Vitamin A 0%	•	Vitamin C 0%
Calcium 0%	•	Iron 0%

˙Percent Daily Values are based on a 2,000 calorie diet. Your daily values may be higher or lower depending on your calorie needs.

	Calories	2,000	2,500
Total Fat	Less than	65g	80g
Sat Fat	Less than	20g	25g
Cholesterol	Less than	300mg	300mg
Sodium	Less than	2,400mg	2,400mg
Potassium		3,500mg	3,500mg
Total Carbohydrate		300g	375g
Dietary Fiber		25g	30g

This label is for black-eyed peas.

1. *Serving size.* Based on the amount most often eaten.
2. *Servings per container.* The number of servings included in the package.
3. *Calories and calories from fat.* "Calories" measures the amount of energy supplied by a food. "Calories from fat" shows the number of fat calories the food supplies.
4. *Fat.* The total amount of fat and the saturated fat included in each serving.
5. *Cholesterol.* The total amount of cholesterol per serving.
6. *Sodium.* The amount of salt per serving.
7. *Potassium.* The amount of potassium per serving.
8. *Carbohydrate.* The total amount of carbohydrate included in each serving, broken down into dietary fiber and sugars.
9. *Protein.* The amount of protein (both in grams and as a percentage of daily value) per serving.

10. *Vitamins and minerals.* Only two vitamins (A and C) and two minerals (calcium and iron) are required on food labels.
11. *Daily value.* Based on a 2,000-calorie meal plan. Your percentage of daily value depends on your total calorie needs per day.

Doing the Math

One gram of fat has nine calories. One gram of either carbohydrate or protein has four calories. To figure the percentage of calories from fat, for example, in a food that contains 100 calories per serving:

3 grams of fat $\times$ 9 calories $=$ 27 calories
27 $\div$ 100 (calories per serving) $=$ 0.27
0.27 $\times$ 100 total calories $=$ 27%

So 27 percent of the calories of one serving come from fat.

Restaurant Labels

The accuracy of many fast-food restaurants' nutrition information is questionable. If you like to eat out, read food labels, choose a menu item that meets your needs, and take care to note how you feel after eating that food. Once you have identified a particular menu item that you enjoy and that seems to regulate your blood sugar, stick with it. For more about eating right in restaurants and on the road, see Chapter 17.

Label Terms

Some foods are claimed to be "light," "cholesterol free," or "low fat." These claims can be used only if they meet the government's definitions.

- *Calorie free.* Less than 5 calories.
- *Cholesterol free.* Less than 2 milligrams of cholesterol and 2 grams or less of saturated fat per serving.
- *Fat free.* Each serving contains less than half a gram of fat.
- *High fiber.* At least 5 grams of fiber.

- *Light* or *lite*. One-third fewer calories or 50 percent less fat; if more than half the calories are from fat, fat content must be reduced by 50 percent or more.
- *Light sodium*. 50 percent less sodium.
- *Low calorie*. 40 calories or less per serving.
- *Low cholesterol*. 20 milligrams or less of cholesterol and 2 grams or less of saturated fat.
- *Low fat*. Less than 3 grams of fat per serving. In calculating the nutritive value in meals, "low fat" means no more than 30 percent of calories from fat.
- *Low saturated fat*. No more than 1 gram of saturated fat per serving and no more than 15 percent of total calories from saturated fat.
- *Low sodium*. 140 milligrams or less of sodium per serving.
- *Reduced* or *less*. 25 percent less of a nutrient than a comparable product.
- *Sugar free*. Less than 0.5 gram of sugar per serving.
- *Very low sodium*. 35 milligrams or less of sodium.

Quick Scan Method for Label Reading

First determine how much of the product is in a single serving. If you generally eat more than the allotted serving amount, you will need to account for the extra amount in your calculations. Compare the given serving size to the amount you will actually consume.

Check the fat content. If it comprises more than 30 percent of the product's total calories, skip it. This food is so high in fat it may throw off your total fat calories for the day. Carbohydrate content will be listed in grams. Choose foods that are high in complex carbohydrates. A food high in simple carbohydrates is high in sugar.

Review the first few ingredients. Since they are listed in order of descending weight, the product is made mostly of these first few ingredients. If they are refined sugars or fat, you want to avoid them. In general, ingredients that have long names and are hard to pronounce are most likely chemical compounds, probably synthetic and best avoided.

When choosing grain products, look for the term "whole grain." For example, "wheat flour" is deceiving: it does not indicate whole-wheat flour. Most flour is made from wheat, but it is generally highly refined, which means the fiber and nutrient-dense parts have been removed. So look for the word "whole" before the ingredient name. Whole-grain products are nutritionally superior. Their natural fiber component is still intact, so they will be digested more slowly and have a lower glycemic response.

17

Restaurant and Travel Tips

ℰating the right foods when you're away from home can be especially challenging. But more and more restaurants are appealing to consumers' health consciousness with new, more nutritious menus. And there are other steps you can take to make road trips more healthful.

Eating Right in Restaurants

Always ask for a nutrition analysis of menu items before you order food in a restaurant. If you can't get a nutrient break-down, you can reduce your risk of eating unexpected calories or too much fat by following a few basic guidelines. Order simple, no-frills items from the menu: perhaps a chicken breast with no skin or gravy, asparagus with no sauce, or whole-grain toast with no butter. Or try bean soup with no bacon, eggs over easy, or salad dressed with balsamic vinegar, lemon, and sea salt.

Fast-Food Restaurants

Many fast-food restaurants have nutrition information posted. It's often in a format similar to the nutrition facts labels on pack-aged foods; see Chapter 16 for a sample label.

Sugar and fat are often hidden in dressings, sauces, bean or meat dishes, soups, and baked goods, adding an unknown num-ber of calories to your meal. For example, as of 1998, the Taco Time chain did not add any fat to its refried beans, while Taco Bell did add fat. Obviously the beans without fat are lower in calories and a healthier choice. You can calculate the calories in beans without fat just as you would count the calories in whole cooked beans.

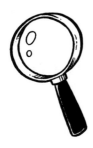 It takes some detective work to find out the number of calories in restaurant items, but it's worth it if you like to eat out. It's the only way to calculate your total caloric intake and count the carbohydrates accurately. If you try to guess, you'll probably underestimate the amounts of fat and sugar (and calories) you consume.

Ordering items with few ingredients makes calculating calories easier. It leaves less room for hidden, high-calorie ingredients to sneak up on you and throw off your blood sugar.

If you eat in fast-food restaurants much, it would be worth purchasing *The Fast Food Guidebook*, published by the Center for Science in the Public Interest (CSPI). This compilation offers nutrition analyses for each of the big fast-food restaurants' menu items.

Center for Science in the Public Interest
1875 Connecticut Ave. NW, Ste. 300
Washington, D.C. 20009-5728

Eating Right on the Road

Take the following nutritional issues into consideration when you travel:
- Changes in meal patterns
- Changes in time zone
- Increased activity
- Decreased activity

Try to stay on the mealtime and medication schedule you are accustomed to at home. If you are traveling for only a short period of time, you may want to eat at the same times you normally do even if they are different from those around you. For example it may be worth it to eat your dinner as scheduled at 6:00 P.M.—even if it is actually 9:00 P.M. where you are. However, if you are traveling for an extended period of time, you will need to adjust to your new time zone or schedule.

TRAVEL CHECKLIST

- Discuss your travel plans with your doctor. If you are traveling out of your time zone, discuss how to handle mealtimes and medication schedules.
- Order extra prescriptions and glucose tabs for emergencies.
- Get a letter from your doctor explaining that you have diabetes and an extra written prescription for your medications.
- Get immunization shots three to four weeks before vacation. Be aware that some shots can affect blood sugar levels.
- Buy snacks to take on flights, on trains, in the car, and in your bag. Nuts and seeds; fruit rollups; protein bars; and aseptic boxes of soy milk, rice milk, and juice all travel well and do not need refrigeration.

ON THE ROAD LIST

- Wear medical identification.
- Keep medication, syringes, and equipment for testing blood sugar in carry-on luggage.
- Take enough medication and medical supplies to last an extra week in case you get stranded or stay longer than planned.
- Have a traveling companion carry some of your medical supplies and emergency sugar source, if possible.
- Inform the airlines and cruise ships in advance that you have diabetes. Most airlines and cruise ships will supply special meals.
- Test your blood sugar more often than usual. Changes in meal patterns, activity levels, and time zones can affect it.

- Always keep snacks and water with you when you are going to be in a situation you can't control (like stuck in traffic).
- Always carry some type of sugar source and protein snacks.

TRAVEL SNACKS

- *Peanuts.* Make your own trail mix with nuts, seeds, and currants.
- *Muesli.* Bring your own whole-grain cereal, premeasured in zip-lock bags. You just add milk and it's ready to eat.
- *Sesame bars.* These high-protein snacks are individually packaged and travel well. They make great emergency snacks when you can't get to a meal.
- *Boxes of milk.* Soy milk, rice milk, and oat milk are all available in aseptic packaging. These little single-serving boxes come with their own straw and do not require refrigeration. They also won't break and don't have lids that might pop off.
- *Fruit rollups.* Buy the ones that are made with real fruits and without food colorings and preservatives.

18

Food Allergies

*F*ood allergies can affect blood sugar regulation. Food reactions are common in the United States. They vary from mild food sensitivity to severe allergies. Food allergies often go undiagnosed because many of their symptoms are the same as the symptoms of blood sugar imbalance.

Eliminating food allergies will improve your immune functioning and overall health and make it easier to identify symptoms related to blood sugar fluctuations. Food allergies are generally a symptom themselves of underlying problems, such as candida, leaky-gut syndrome, heavy-metal poisoning, parasites, or viral infection. Generally the underlying condition can be treated and the food allergies will diminish or be completely under control within a year.

Symptoms and Diagnosis

Keeping a food diary will provide the first clues of food allergies. Many of the symptoms of food allergies are similar to those that affect the nervous system when blood sugar drops or rises dramatically. Food allergy symptoms include the following:

anxiety	fatigue
confusion	headaches
delusions	insomnia
depression	irritability
dizziness	poor concentration
drowsiness	poor memory
faintness	weakness

Causes and Treatment

An allergic reaction is an inflammation response to a foreign substance, such as a food or an inhalant. The body's defense mechanisms respond by identifying and trying to eliminate the antigen. It is your body's way of protecting you from foreign substances.

Eliminating Food Allergies

Common allergenic foods are wheat, dairy products, and corn. The foods that we tend to eat a lot of are generally the culprits. Food additives, agricultural pesticides and herbicides (such as sulfites, MSG, BHA, and BHT), as well as synthetic sweeteners (such as aspartame and saccharin) can all cause reactions.

Purchase whole, organic, unprocessed foods. Avoid packaged foods made with food colorings and preservatives.

Identifying Allergies

Several tests are used to diagnose food allergies: elimination trials, skin-prick tests, and blood tests. These tests will result in a variety of responses. There are four recognized types of allergic or hypersensitivity reactions.

Type I immediate-onset allergic reaction is the true, classic allergic response when there is an Immunoglobin E–mediated response to a food. It is characterized by the binding of IgE antibodies to a specific antigen. When IgE-sensitized white blood cells contact an antigen, they release a barrage of chemical defenses. Each has its own destructive actions. They include the following inflammatory agents:

- Lysosomal enzymes, which digest and destroy tissue
- Histamine, which causes leakage from capillaries and produces tissue swelling
- Toxic free radicals, which destroy cellular membranes, accelerate the aging process, and contribute to arteriosclerosis and arthritis

- Arachidonic acid, which is converted into the prostaglandin-2 hormone series (PGE-2), which stimulates the release of leukotrienes (See Chapter 3 of *Optimal Wellness*, a book cited in Suggested Reading Materials in the Appendix.)
- Kinin and bradykinin-like substances, which are destructive inflammation catalysts

Type 2 delayed-onset reactions are the allergylike responses that involve the IgA antibodies and cellular T lymphocytes. A delayed reaction to eating a food could take up to several days to show symptoms. These are largely diagnosed by conventional skin tests.

Elimination Trials

When you suspect a food is an allergen, try avoiding it for several weeks. Write down what you eat and how you feel in your meal plan record before you eliminate the food, then during the elimination, and again when you add it back into the diet. Diaries are a helpful method for identifying physical and mental changes in your health. Most allergies have a root cause, such as candida or toxicity. Once the underlying cause of the allergy has been eliminated, most people find that they are able to eat the formerly allergenic food. Introduce each food back into the diet one at a time. Rotate each one slowly into the diet. Eating those foods occasionally, meaning only a few times a week, will reduce the chance of recurring responses.

Clinical Laboratory Tests

Several tests are available for identifying food allergies. The elimination diet is the least invasive and least expensive route, but if you are very ill and suspect allergies, ask your doctor for immediate testing. If your doctor is not accustomed to checking for allergies, find an expert in your area or share the following addresses with your doctor. Generally your physician will be able to arrange for a blood draw and the shipment to the lab.

Labs that do allergy testing:

Immuno Laboratories
1620 West Oakland Park Blvd.
Fort Lauderdale, FL 33311
(305) 486-4500
(800) 231-9197

Meridian Valley Clinical Laboratory
24030 132nd Ave. SE
Kent, WA 98042
(206) 631-8922
(800) 234-6825

MetaMetrics Inc.
Medical Research Laboratory
3000 Northwoods Pkwy., Ste. 150
Northcross, GA 30071
(404) 446-5483
(800) 221-4640

National Bio Technology Laboratory
3212 Northeast 125th St., Ste. D
Seattle, WA 98125-9826
(206) 363-6006
(800) 846-6285

Serammune Physicians Lab
1890 Preston White Dr., 2nd Fl.
Reston, VA 22091
(703) 758-0610
(800) 553-5472

Further Resources

For more information about food allergies and treatment and about the multiple conditions that predispose us to food allergies, read *Optimal Wellness* by Ralph Golan, M.D. (Ballantine, 1995). This book should be in every home. Dr. Golan explains in lay terms complex overlapping conditions like liver toxicity, adrenal exhaustion, yeast overgrowth, toxic bowel, and hypoglycemia and how these underlying conditions can lead to disease states. He also defines the steps necessary to heal through nutrition, supplementation, and detoxification.

For a free newsletter about food allergies called *Allergy Alert*, contact Dr. Sally Rockwell. Dr. Rockwell is a nutritionist and expert in treating food allergies and candida.

Sally J. Rockwell, C.N., Ph.D.
P.O. Box 31065
Seattle, WA 98103
(206) 547-1814
Fax (206) 547-7696
E-mail: docrock@accessone.com
Website: www.arxc.com/doctors/rockwell.htm

19

....

Artificial Sweeteners

*A*n estimated 70 percent of the sweeteners or sugars added to beverages and processed foods are artificial, not natural. Many new artificial (synthetic) sweeteners are being marketed directly to people with diabetes. The ad campaigns and product labels promote these sweeteners as "free foods." The producers encourage mass consumption, in unlimited quantities and combinations.

As people with diabetes accept these additives and the food products that contain them into their daily diets, many are experiencing subtle to severe negative reactions. This can be attributed to many factors—including the other ingredients in the product, such as dextrose or lactose buffers, which may exacerbate blood glucose.

These products are still so new that there is little educational material or nutritional information available to consumers regarding their safety and efficacy. Synthetic sweeteners are genetically manipulated food components. They are not natural in any way. Large corporations are making enormous profits from the sale of these products and are promoting them without long-term studies or safety screening. The Food and Drug Administration often allows products like these onto our market shelves due to pressure by lobbyists, only to pull them a few years later as the effects begin to surface. Already we are experiencing a backlash of health problems from the genetically altered foods that are now part of our food supply.

Aspartame, the sweetener whose trade name is Nutra-Sweet™, has exhibited neurotoxic (brain-damaging) potential. The FDA has been analyzing aspartame's potential to exacerbate preexisting capacity for mental retardation, brain lesioning, and central nervous system cancers in animals.

These are not light accusations. The list of side effects from aspartame, as well as other synthetic sweeteners on the market today, is long. Elevated cholesterol levels, diarrhea, metabolic disturbances, dizziness, nausea, testicular atrophy, decreased fuel oxidation, and seizures have all been directly associated with the use of synthetic sweeteners.

Artificial Sweeteners and the Little People

Artificial sweeteners are chemicals that wreak havoc on the workers of our metabolism. These chemicals interfere with blood sugar storage in the liver, hunger messages, cellular division, sleep patterns, and many other biological systems. The little people have been trained for thousands of years to do their delicate jobs in a very specific fashion, dealing with the breakdown and absorption of whole foods. When they are given chemicals as food, it increases the cleanup work they have to do to get rid of these indigestible materials and it keeps the immune system workers busy. When your immune system is tied up on a big job, it can't protect you from invaders and improper cell division. Your body becomes susceptible to viral and bacterial attack and cancer development. The little people hate synthetic sweeteners. It makes their jobs a whole lot easier if you eat smaller quantities of natural sugars that they are familiar with—especially if you eat those sugars with a meal so they are absorbed as slowly as possible.

The Effects of Artificial Sweeteners

Artificial sweeteners have many side effects. Here we look at just a few: blood sugar imbalance, dehydration and electrolyte imbalance, reduced absorption of nutrients, and caffeine complications.

Blood Sugar Imbalance

Some sweeteners cause a rise in blood sugar; others cause a drop. This appears to be a result of amino acid metabolites. Certain amino acids are known to stimulate insulin secretion, thus dropping blood sugar levels, while others stimulate the secretion of glucagon (stored blood sugar), which raises blood sugar levels.

Dehydration and Electrolyte Imbalance

Overuse of any of the synthetic sweeteners has the potential to cause runny stools, which can lead to dehydration, which in turn raises blood sugar concentration in the blood. Mannitol, in fact, is a baby laxative that causes runny stool, diarrhea, and gas. Dehydration is especially prevalent in people who consume sodas rather than water on a regular basis.

Reduced Nutrient Absorption

Irritated bowels and constant mucous coating in the intestinal tract hinder the absorption of nutrients.

Caffeine Complications

Many of these synthetic products, such as cocoa and cola drinks, also contain caffeine. The caffeine causes a second set of problems that overlay the previously mentioned ones. Caffeine has a laxative effect, which hinders nutrient absorption and electrolyte maintenance. Caffeine also interferes with hunger signals. A lack of clear biofeedback to the brain as to energy levels and reserves is risky to the health of diabetics.

The History of Artificial Sweeteners

Artificial sweeteners have not been tested on humans over a long period of time. We are the first generation to test these products. People with compromised metabolisms, such as those with diabetes, should not be the guinea pigs for this global corporate experiment.

Chemical corporations make these products and promote their sale and use in the media and through our health professionals. It is important that we be informed consumers, particularly where our health is at risk.

The NutraSweet Story

Aspartame's introduction to the market was filled with excitement. Here was a palatable product composed only of substances normally found in food: aspartic acid, phenylalanine, and methanol. It was proposed that even high doses of such safe ingredients would have relatively few side effects.

But then the Centers for Disease Control (CDC) published results of a study based on passive surveillance of consumer-initiated complaints associated with aspartame-containing food products. Several hundred subjects completed a CDC questionnaire about their side effects. Complaints were as follows:

- headaches
- central nervous system disorders
- mood changes
- insomnia
- seizures
- gastrointestinal tract disorders
- abdominal pain
- nausea
- diarrhea
- gynecological symptoms
- irregular menses

The CDC's report concluded that the "highest priority for any future investigation might be in the neurological-behavioral area."

It appears that the amino acid phenylalanine causes a rise in blood sugar for some people. As phenylalanine breaks down in the digestive tract to tyrosine, it signals the liver to dump its glycogen (stored sugar), which then enters the bloodstream. If you are noticing dramatic blood sugar fluctuations after ingesting synthetic sweeteners, stop using them.

Lessons from Our Past

Concern about the health risks of synthetic sweeteners stem from their track record. Cyclamates were approved by the FDA in the 1950s and sold in food products ranging from chewing gum to soft drinks. At that time, 175 million Americans were consuming significant doses of what they considered to be a safe food additive. Cyclamates were removed from the market in 1969 because they were found to cause bladder cancer in rats.

America's love affair with new products keeps a constant flow of synthetic products into the market, but there are just as many products pulled from the shelves in any given year as there are new ones introduced. The FDA has concluded that some chemical sweeteners may not be carcinogenic alone but may enhance the effect of other cancer-causing substances.

Current and common acceptance, FDA approval, and extensive marketing do not necessarily make a product safe. You must ultimately decide whether you are willing to risk their health effects. Be advised that because children's brains are in constant development, the neurotoxic effects of synthetic sweeteners and their by-products may have a more profound impact on children.

Many types of products contain synthetic sweeteners:

- low-calorie whipped topping
- sugar-free hard candy
- sugar-free ice cream
- sugar-free gum
- sugar-free flavored gelatin or Jell-O
- sugar-free cocoa
- low-calorie pancake syrup
- sugar-free soda pop
- sugar-free pudding
- low-calorie salad dressing

Types of Artificial Sweeteners

Altimate

The as yet unapproved sweetener altimate is two thousand times sweeter than sugar. It is made from the amino acids L-aspartic acid and L-alanine and 2,2,4,4-tetramethylthieanyl amine. A petition seeking approval for altimate was submitted to the FDA in 1986.

Aspartame

The dipeptide sweetener aspartame has the trade names NutraSweet and Equal. It is a synthetic compound prepared from aspartic acid, phenylalanine, and methanol. This amino acid compound contains four calories per gram and is two hundred times sweeter than natural sugar.

The FDA reports several neurotoxic effects of aspartame. Both glutamic acid and aspartic acid may induce lesions in the hypothalamus of the brain, which can lead to Parkinson's disease, and at higher doses other portions of the brain and the retina may be permanently damaged. Aspartic acid, phenylalanine, and methanol are all metabolic breakdown products of aspartame. Methanol is known to damage the retina.

In 1988, the Mexican government stopped soda and food processors from using the word "nutra" in the brand name because it was misleading. The Mexicans also required labeling to carry the following warning: "This product should not be used by individuals who are allergic to phenylalanine. Consumption by pregnant women and children less than seven years is not recommended. Users should follow a balanced diet. Consumption by those with diabetes must be authorized by a physician."

The CDC warns that some individuals may be more sensitive to aspartame's effects than others. It lowers acidity of urine and therefore reportedly makes the urinary tract more susceptible to infection. People with phenylketonuria (PKU) must avoid phenylalanine.

Acesulfame Potassium

Also know as Sweet One (and Acesulfame K), acesulfame potassium received approval from the FDA in 1988 and is marketed under the name Sunette. It is 130 to 200 times sweeter than sugar. It is used in chewing gum, dry beverage mixes, confections, canned fruit, gelatins, puddings, and custards and as a tabletop sweetener. Animal studies that show that this product stimulates tumor growth have been debated.

Cyclamates

Cyclamates are thirty times sweeter than sugar, water soluble, and heat stable. They were removed from the food market in 1969 because they were found to cause bladder cancer in rats. At that time 175 million Americans were swallowing cyclamates in significant doses in many products, ranging from chewing gum to soft drinks. A petition to reapprove the use of cyclamates is currently under review by the FDA.

L-Sugars

L-sugars are chemical sweeteners that act and taste like table sugar but will not metabolize. They are chemically arranged as a mirror image of regular table sugar. The problem with such chemical products is in how the body recognizes these foreign substances. L-sugars are not yet considered acceptable alternatives.

Maltitol

Maltitol, a corn powder derivative, is advertised as safe for diabetics. It is digested in the intestinal tract, not in the stomach. It can cause gastric disturbances such as bloating, gas, and diarrhea. If you try a product containing maltitol, closely observe its effects on your blood sugar levels. If you notice blood sugar increases with its consumption, avoid this product.

Saccharin

Saccharin is a coal tar derivative found in the product Sweet 'n Low and in many colas and sodas. It is the oldest synthetic/non-nutritive sweetener in the U.S. food supply. First synthesized accidentally in 1879, it was originally intended to be used solely as an antiseptic agent in the treatment of bladder infections. When researchers discovered it is 300 times sweeter than natural sugar, they began to use it as a substitute for sugar in canned vegetables and beverages.

Saccharin is synthesized from toluene and has a bitter aftertaste. It was used with cyclamates in the experiments that led to the ban on cyclamates. After the FDA banned cyclamates in 1970, saccharin was the only nonnutritive sweetener approved for use in the United States. It is now on the FDA's top priority list to retest for mutagenic, subacute, and reproductive effects. Studies show a link to bladder cancer, so it is best to minimize the use of all saccharin products.

Sorbitol

Sorbitol has half the calories and half the sweetness of table sugar. Because sorbitol is found naturally in plants, it may be considered natural, but it is usually manufactured commercially.

Thaumatin

Thaumatin is a combination of sweet-tasting fruit proteins currently used to flavor chewing gum.

Xylitol

At one time extracted from the birch tree, xylitol is now made from waste products of the pulp industry. It has about one-fourth the calories of sugar. The FDA's preliminary reports cited it as a possible cancer-causing agent, and it has proved carcinogenic in animal studies. It is reported to have a diuretic effect and is linked to bladder stones, tumors, and liver anomalies.

Reasons to Avoid Artificial Sweeteners

Some synthetic sweeteners increase the incidence of bladder cancer and tumor development. (Anderson 1979, Crapo 1989) There is a significant increase in the risk of cancer when several synthetic sweeteners are combined in the diet. (Crapo 1989) There is evidence that phenylalanine found in diet drinks is the cause of blood sugar spikes in people with diabetes. (Haire-Joshu 1992)

The Center for Science in the Public Interest has published a list of synthetic sweeteners and a host of possible side effects. They include elevated cholesterol levels, diarrhea, metabolic disturbances, dizziness, nausea, testicular atrophy, decreased fuel oxidation, and seizures. (Bantle et al. 1992, Collings 1989, Miller and Frattali 1989)

Some synthetic sweeteners are not only potentially toxic but appetite stimulants. Far from decreasing appetite (as once thought), they have caused a 10 to 15 percent increase in food intake in rats given a saccharin solution rather than water. (Horwitz et al. 1988, Porikos and Koopmans 1988)

The extensive array of synthetic sweeteners and the products that contain them are being aggressively marketed to the diabetic population. (Warshaw and Powers 1993) Current studies on the adverse health effects caused by overuse of synthetic sweeteners have not yet been considered in diabetic dietary protocols. (Franz et al. 1994) Testing each of the individual sweeteners for carcinogenicity and its potential as a hepatic glycogen-release stimulant is vital. Long-term risk assessment for individual and combination ingestion of alternative sweeteners is necessary before safety can be determined. In the meantime, it may be advisable to limit your intake. Try substituting a natural sweetener such as stevia root.

FDA Assessment

The Food and Drug Administration currently approves all of the sweeteners listed in this chapter unless otherwise stated. But research has uncovered too many questions about their safety and efficacy for us to recommend them to any degree. They are not whole foods or natural foods—they are not even real foods. They are not organic and they are certainly not kosher, since they have been genetically altered.

ADA Policy Statement

The official recommendation from the American Diabetes Association for synthetic sweeteners is outdated in that it still lists these food products as free foods. This was based on the concept that they contain no calories or carbohydrates, but we know now that they can still raise blood sugar levels through other mechanisms.

All artificial sweeteners have a host of side effects. Some increase the risk of diseases such as cancer, while others actually affect blood sugar levels. Blood sugar fluctuations are experienced in varying degrees depending on the chemical components of the sweetener and the individual consuming it.

20

The Effects of Caffeine, Alcohol, and Cigarettes

*H*abits such as smoking and drinking coffee or alcohol have a profound effect on your health if they become part of your daily or even weekly schedule. When you're trying to break them, it helps to be aware of the ways these bad habits affect the diabetes process.

Caffeine

Coffee, black tea, soft drinks, chocolate, cocoa, and many prescription and over-the-counter medications contain caffeine. The feelings of alertness and energy come from their effects on the nervous system and the stimulation of the adrenal glands.

Caffeine affects diabetes through many actions. For example:

- It stimulates cortisol and adrenaline from the adrenal glands, which elevate blood sugar levels.
- It causes nervousness and decreased coping ability, which may hinder a diabetic person's handling of insulin and medications.
- It can cause urinary loss of calcium, magnesium, biotin, and inositol, which people with diabetes are inherently deficient in.
- It disrupts fat metabolism, raises blood cholesterol, and increases electrolyte loss, which all exacerbate heart disease.
- It can cause sleep disruption and insomnia, which exacerbate depression.

Alcohol

If you have high blood pressure or high triglyceride levels or if you are in doubt as to whether or not consuming alcohol is safe for you, check with your doctor. Drink alcohol only when your blood sugar level is well controlled. All alcohol is high in calories and impairs your faculties and decision-making processes—including your ability to monitor your blood sugar. Use alcohol sparingly because it is so quickly metabolized that it can easily imbalance blood sugar levels. It will also displace the healthful, nutritious foods that you need to eat.

Drinking alcohol has the following effects:

- It profoundly depresses production of white blood cells.
- It elevates blood cholesterol, triglyceride, and uric acid levels.
- It elevates blood pressure.
- It increases the risk of atherosclerosis.
- It exacerbates psoriasis, which is already associated with diabetes.
- It inhibits liver function.

If you drink at all, drink moderately and follow these guidelines:

- Don't have more than two drinks a week.
- Consume alcohol only with food.
- Calculate alcohol as carbohydrates in the exchange system.
- Avoid sugary drinks such as wine coolers, hard cider, Irish cream, and cordials.
- Avoid high-sugar mixers such as Coke, grenadine syrup, and concentrated fruit juice.

Cigarettes

Cigarette smoking has a wide range of negative effects that worsen the diabetic condition. Fortunately, many of the effects are reversed when you stop smoking.

Smoking cigarettes (or cigars) has the following effects, among others:

- It increases the load of free radicals, which suppresses the immune system.
- It is a potent risk factor in atherosclerosis, for which people with diabetes are already at risk.
- It increases the overall risk of death by 70 percent.
- It causes vitamin C deficiency.
- It stimulates the adrenal secretion of cortisol and adrenaline, which causes low blood sugar and hypertension.
- It increases cortisol production, which decreases the uptake of tryptophan, which decreases the production of serotonin, which leads to depression.
- It increases the level of cadmium and lead in the blood, which leads to kidney stones.
- It is associated with dramatic increases in periodontal disease, particularly damage to the surface cells of the gums.

21

Oral Health

$\mathcal{D}$iabetes can create changes in the oral environment that make it especially important to pay attention to this area of the body. Only 2 percent of the population is cavity free; the statistics are not in our favor from the beginning. And the beginning starts before we are born, so the importance of good nutrition in all life stages of growth and development can never be overemphasized. At the other end of the spectrum is periodontal disease, an insidious process of gum-tissue infection and consequent breakdown of tissue support that is actually responsible for the loss of more teeth than decay is in people over age thirty-five.

The good news is that the signs and symptoms are detectable and generally controllable, maintainable, and even correctable with good oral hygiene, regular checkups, and proper balanced nutrition.

The Periodontal Process

The mechanics of tooth decay and periodontal disease are easy to understand: Sugars on teeth lead to the formation of sticky plaque. This increases acid-forming bacteria, which results in tooth decay. The same bacteria that invade the tooth are responsible for periodontal disease, a term used to encompass the stages of breakdown in periodontal tissues surrounding and supporting the teeth.

Bacteria on teeth + Predisposing hereditary factor +
  Ineffective cleaning = Gingivitis

= Increase of inflammation of tissues and increase of
 bacteria + Formation of tartar or calculus (calcium
 deposits)
= Destruction of surrounding tissues (ligamental fibers and
 bone
= Pocket formation
= Periodontal disease and further destruction until the tooth
 becomes loose and exfoliates (falls out)

Periodontal disease can be isolated in one or two areas, or the entire mouth can be involved. Left unchecked and untreated, the entire process becomes circular.

How Does Diabetes Affect Oral Health?

Along with a diagnosis of diabetes comes the possibility of a number of additional oral problems. Every disease process manifests orally at some stage of development. Many nutritional signs and symptoms are revealed in an oral exam. Therefore, your dentist or dental hygienist can be an important part of your team of health-care professionals in recognizing factors that need attention. Some examples follow:

General fatigue from diabetes can cause a range of effects, including a reduction in exercise, which can lead to reduced blood circulation, emotional depression, and stress. These and other factors can further deplete the capacity of the immune system. Symptoms of this can be directly observed in the mouth.

Stress, as we are learning, can cause a wide range of responses on a physical as well as psychological and emotional levels. Orally, the body sometimes responds to stress through a condition called *bruxism*, or the grinding of teeth. This can lead to tooth sensitivity or possibly pain in the jaw or headaches from the stresses on the temporomandibular joint (TMJ) and surrounding musculature.

Further conditions—such as an increased vulnerability to gingivitis, canker sores, cold sores (herpes simplex), or candida albicans (thrush or yeast infection)—are all possible with diabetes if the immune system is overstressed (See Chapter 23 for more about candida.)

Changes in oral tissues related to vitamin deficiencies are often observed, particularly at the corners of the mouth and the tongue. This can be due to lack of intake and/or lack of absorption.

Certain medications associated with any number of the conditions related to diabetes can cause severe vomiting, the effects of which will eventually manifest as the erosion of tooth enamel at the gum line. Still other medications, or the disease itself, can cause a reduction of salivary flow, reducing the ability to digest starches as well as restricting the natural cleansing action of the mouth.

Although we know a great deal about the mechanisms of tooth decay and periodontal disease, no cure exists to date. Prevention is our best defense.

Personal Oral Hygiene

The most important tool for preventing periodontal disease is your personal oral hygiene. Oral bacteria will multiply to a destructive level in any given mouth over twelve to twenty-four hours. Some mouths are more resistant, due to a variety of factors, but the basic rule is to brush your teeth at least twice a day and floss at least once. Floss in the evening to dislodge food particles that might otherwise rest on the teeth overnight. After brushing and/or flossing, always rinse thoroughly with water to remove what has been dislodged. Run the brush gently over your tongue, an area that harbors a lot of bacteria. Be sure to change your toothbrush often (at least every six months), both to maintain its shape and to reduce bacterial contamination.

Regular Dental Checkups

For all the reasons mentioned here as well as the need for tooth checkups and cleanings, dental visits should be made as frequently as deemed necessary by your dental team. Generally an exam every six months is sufficient. Always inform your dentist of any medical changes, including new or discontinued medications. You may need more frequent visits or special tools for adequate home care.

Special Tools

Tools such as the Sonicare toothbrush, floss holders, stimulators for gum tissues, irrigators for air pockets, and special rinses to reduce bacterial levels as well as protect eroded enamel may be appropriate for you. Ask questions of your dentist and hygienist to be sure your needs are met.

Oral Health and Your Meal Plan

Fresh whole foods and pure water are the building blocks to oral health. A well-balanced meal plan designed to meet your needs is essential for healing any disease process.

Sugar

Clearly, the less sugar in your diet, the less possibility for tooth decay. This includes all of the simple sugars and is especially true of foods that are sticky and stay on the teeth for a while.

Timing and Types of Foods

Both the timing of food intake and the particular foods eaten can have a direct effect on bacterial growth. Frequent sipping of soft drinks or continual snacking will maintain oral acid at peak levels without allowing time for oral pH to return to normal. Whole foods such as legumes, grains, and vegetables help raise the pH from an acidic level, thus reducing the possibility of caries (cavities). Foods that promote salivary flow are highly beneficial. If you still don't produce enough saliva, your dentist can recommend a salivary enhancer. Homeopathic, Chinese, and Ayurvedic medicines all have natural stimulants that work to promote the flow of saliva as well.

Physical Signs of Nutrient Deficiencies

As mentioned, many physical symptoms of nutrient deficiencies are visible upon oral inspection by your dentist or dental hygienist. Physical symptoms may warrant clinical tests to confirm a deficiency. Tests can help determine whether the deficiency is caused by malabsorption or lack of intake. After evaluating these tests, your dentist, doctor, naturopath, or nutritionist may recommend vitamin and mineral supplements. This is another area where the team of medical experts you assembled in Chapter 10 can serve you well.

22

Phytochemicals and Blood Sugar Regulation

The prefix *phyto* means plant. There are natural components in plant foods called phytochemicals that have been medically proved to help regulate blood sugar. Some of the best are found in bitter melon, fenugreek, licorice, holy basil, and garlic.

Bitter Melon

Bitter melon (Momordica charantia) also known as balsam pear, is a tropical Asian fruit. This green, long, bumpy fruit looks somewhat like a cucumber. The juice of the unripe fruit contains phytochemicals whose medicinal properties are helpful to people with diabetes. For example, charantin is a chemical composed of several steroids that reduces blood sugar more efficiently than the oral drug tolbutamide. Drinking just two ounces of bitter melon juice each day has been effective in reducing blood sugar levels.

A Replacement for Insulin?

Bitter melon contains the insulinlike polypeptide-P, which lowers blood sugar levels when injected. Since it has fewer side effects than insulin, it shows promise as an insulin replacement therapy. (Welihinda et al. 1982)

Fenugreek

Fenugreek (Trigonella foenumgraecum) seeds are sold as a spice or can be purchased in the produce department of the grocery store. They contain alkaloid trigonelline, nicotinic acid, and

FENUGREEK SEEDS (MAGNIFIED)

coumarin. The seeds can be eaten raw to reduce fasting blood sugar and improve glucose tolerance.

Garlic

Garlic (Allium sativum) contains the medicinally active oil allicin. Garlic's effects on blood glucose control lie in its ability to reduce the breakdown of insulin, which increases its availability. The allicin oils break down and become much less potent when cooked. Chew them raw or add them to dips, salsa, fresh vegetables, juices, or salad dressing.

Raw garlic is an effective broad-spectrum antimicrobial. Its properties are effective against:

staph	candida
strep	roundworm
bacillus	hookworm
e. coli	influenza
salmonella	

The cardiovascular benefits of raw or cooked garlic include the following:

- It decreases triglyceride levels.
- It decreases cholesterol levels (total and LDL).
- It raises HDL cholesterol.
- It lowers blood pressure.
- It prevents excessive blood-clot formation.

Raw garlic may not taste great to some people. The salad dressing on page 248 makes a delicious disguise for it. Add as much garlic as you like.

Holy Basil

Holy basil is known as tulsi in India and bai gaprao in Thailand. Many Hindus grow this revered plant in their homes. Experimental studies reported that leaf extract of ocimum sanctum and ocimum album (holy basil) had a hypoglycemic affect. These findings suggest that basil leaves may be an adjunct to dietary therapy and drug treatment in mild to moderate noninsulin-dependent diabetes. (Agrawal et al. 1996)

Licorice

Licorice (Glycyrrhiza glabra) root enhances the mucosal lining of the digestive tract. It is used as a tea to prevent gastrointestinal inflammation and ulcers, to protect the liver, for its antimicrobial activity (against staph, strep, and candida), for menopausal symptoms, and to help normalize blood pressure. Licorice root is also used topically on oral and genital herpes lesions to speed healing and reduce pain.

Garlic Ginger Dressing

....

6 cloves raw peeled garlic

2-inch piece of fresh gingerroot, peeled

3 tablespoons balsamic vinegar

½ lemon, seeded and with outer yellow layer of peel
   removed

½ orange, seeded and with outer orange layer of peel
   removed

1 tablespoon flaxseed oil

Add all ingredients to a food processor or blender and blend
for twenty seconds. Serve as a dip or salad dressing. It's also delicious over potatoes, yams, sweet potatoes, cooked carrots, cold
bean salads, lentil salads, and tomato slices.

23

Candida Yeast Overgrowth

$\int$ince people with diabetes often have high blood sugar, they are candidates for **candida** yeast overgrowth and should be aware of the symptoms. Overuse of antibiotics, long-term use of birth control pills, and a high-sugar "junk food" diet over time can all reduce the number of the good, healthful bacteria in the gut and contribute to candida overgrowth.

Symptoms and Disorders

Candida infections cause a host of physical symptoms and disorders.

- menstrual problems, premenstrual tension
- vaginitis
- prostatitis
- loss of libido
- cravings for sugar, bread, alcohol, and yeasty foods
- sensitivity to perfumes, tobacco, and chemical odors
- recurrent digestive problems, especially constipation, abdominal pain, diarrhea, gas, or bloating
- skin conditions such as hives, psoriasis, or other chronic skin rashes
- headaches
- muscle pain or weakness and joint pains
- extreme fatigue or lethargy
- depression, moodiness, inability to concentrate
- fungal infections of the finger or toenails or jock itch
- respiratory symptoms
- hyperactivity

Defining Organisms

Yeasts are single-cell fungi and are similar to molds. You will find the terms *fungi*, *yeast*, and *molds* used interchangeably in literature on the subject.

Beneficial Bacteria

Healthy bacteria—such as the lactobacillus acidophilus and bifidus bacteria—colonize in the large intestine to a great extent and the small intestine to a lesser degree. There they aid in the digestive process by helping to break down undigested food particles and synthesize the B vitamins and vitamin K.

Bad Bacteria

Candida albicans normally inhabits the intestines in small colonies. Candida becomes a problem only when there is an overgrowth, which throws off the delicate balance between these symbiotic organisms.

Diagnosing Candida Overgrowth

Before assuming you have a candida problem, get a professional opinion based on a careful history, physical examination, and clinical lab test results. This is important because many other disorders can cause similar symptoms.

If you have symptoms of candida albicans overgrowth, you should see a medical doctor, naturopathic physician, or nutritionist who is familiar with candida. A stool or blood test will determine the degree of overgrowth. Most clinical labs offer these tests. If your medical center does not, your doctor can send your blood or stool sample to another lab.

Causes of Candida Imbalance

There are many reasons why candida runs wild. Here are the major ones. *Broad-spectrum antibiotics* are powerful germ killers and tend to wipe out entire colonies of healthful bacteria. Once these good bacteria are gone, they leave room for the hardier yeast, such as candida, to take over. Just add sugar and watch them grow. Uncontrolled diabetes and high blood sugar levels create the ideal environment for yeast to grow like crazy.

Birth control pills, *steroids*, and many *medications* reduce B-vitamin levels, which also reduces the defense against candida. If you are taking birth control pills, it is important to take a multivitamin with the RDA of each of the B vitamins, especially B_6.

Pregnancy and *premenstrual phase* increase progesterone and exacerbate candida growth (as do birth control pills).

Sugar and *simple carbohydrates* feed the yeast, causing rapid growth. Carbohydrates break down quickly into sugars in the bloodstream, providing food for the candida to thrive. Diets full of simple carbohydrates such as pasta, white breads, and sugars also contribute to nutrient deficiencies, which play a role in the downward health spiral of the yeast overgrowth.

The Allergy Connection

The liver is the main organ of detoxification in the body. If it gets overloaded with alcohol, caffeine, high-fat foods, or drugs (prescription or recreational), it can't properly detoxify the toxins produced by the candida fungus. By eliminating these "liver loaders," you can speed the treatment and elimination of candida.

Candida keeps the immune system busy working on cleaning the yeast out of the body. If the immune system is overburdened, allergies can develop. Without the keen inspection of the immune system, the body sees certain foods and/or pollens as foreign invaders and reacts allergically. This is why people with diabetes and hypoglycemia often have food allergies.

Treatments for Candida

There are several effective treatments, among them grapefruit seed extract, garlic, nystatin, and caprylic acid in various combinations. It is important that you work with a medical professional who has treated candida patients successfully. Diabetes must be well controlled throughout treatment, with special attention to keeping blood sugar levels within a healthy range. It is also helpful to replace the good bacteria (such as acidophilus and bifidus) with supplements or with food that contains live cultures, like yogurt. When candida has been present for a while, the treatment will often be more effective with nutrient supplementation. It is important to purchase only high-quality supplements. See the list of recommended brands in the Resources section of the Appendix and see Chapter 7 for tips on shopping for vitamins.

Avoiding a Recurrence

To keep candida infections from coming back, follow these simple guidelines.

- Maintain a healthy internal environment for good bacteria with foods or supplements that contain live cultures of acidophilus and bifidus.
- Drink plenty of water.
- Eat high-fiber foods such as legumes, vegetables, and whole grains.
- Keep blood sugar levels in control.
- Avoid sugary foods, fruits, fruit juices, alcohol, and sweet drinks.
- Reduce dairy intake. In severe cases, avoid dairy products completely. They contain the natural sugar lactose, which feeds the candida.

Part IV

༺

Appendixes

Glossary

AA (arachidonic acid)   A long-chain omega-6 fatty acid that contains twenty carbon atoms and four unsaturations ($C20:4n-6$). Found mainly in animal products, AA is the main precursor to series 2 eicosanoids, which constrict blood vessels and quicken blood clotting.

adipose cells   Fat-storing cells. Adipose tissue is fatty tissue composed of a quantity of adipose cells.

alimentary canal   See *gastrointestinal tract*.

amino acids   The basic building blocks of proteins. There are twenty-two amino acids.

antigen A substance, such as food, mold, or pollen, that elicits an immune response.

antioxidants   Chemicals that stop the loss of electrons to free radicals, thereby preventing cellular damage. Common natural antioxidants include vitamins C and E and beta-carotene. (See also *free radicals*.)

arteries   The vessels that carry blood away from the heart. All arteries except the pulmonary artery carry oxygenated blood. (See also *veins*.)

arterioles   The small arteries that are responsible for regulating blood flow into the capillaries.

arteriosclerosis   Diseases characterized by thickening and loss of elasticity of arterial walls.

atherogenic   Relating to or producing degenerative changes in artery walls.

atherosclerosis   A form of arteriosclerosis in which fatty deposits (plaques) form inside the linings of arteries and interfere with the flow of blood. (See also *plaque.*)

BG (blood glucose concentration)   Blood glucose (or blood sugar) is the primary fuel for all cells of the body. People with diabetes usually have fasting BG values in the range of 70 to 120 milligrams per deciliter of blood. BG levels rise in people with untreated diabetes.

brittle diabetes   A diabetic condition characterized by little or no production of insulin, along with extreme increases in blood sugar even when small amounts of food are eaten.

calorie   An energy unit. A single calorie is the amount of heat needed to increase the temperature of one gram of water by one degree centigrade.

candida   A yeast whose overgrowth is a common side effect of high levels of blood sugar. Often referred to as bacteria or fungus.

capillaries   The smallest blood vessels, formed from a single layer of endothelial cells. Capillary blood is blood removed from microscopic vessels near the skin's surface (for example, finger-puncture blood).

carbohydrate   A carbohydrate (CHO) molecule is a chain of two or more sugar molecules. Carbohydrates can be simple or complex. Simple carbohydrates are simple sugar molecules: the monosaccharides (glucose, fructose, and galactose) and the disaccharides (sucrose, maltose, and lactose). Complex carbohydrates, or polysaccharides, are starch molecules built out of many sugar units. Healthful sources of complex carbohydrates are legumes, grains, fruits, and vegetables.

carcinogenic   Known to increase cancer risk or to cause cancer directly. For example, cigarettes are carcinogenic.

cardiovascular system   The heart (cardio) and blood vessels (vascular).

catecholamines   The endocrine hormones adrenaline (also called epinephrine) and norepinephrine. These neurotransmitters regulate functions in glucose metabolism, such as the breakdown of muscle and liver glycogen to glucose and the inhibition of insulin release from the pancreas. They also facilitate the breakdown of fatty acids as an alternate fuel source. (See also *neurotransmitter*.)

cellular respiration   A metabolic process in which cells take in molecular oxygen, organic substances are oxidized, free energy is released, and the cells give off carbon dioxide, water, and other oxidized products. (See also *mitochondria*.)

CHO   The abbreviation for carbohydrate. (See also *carbohydrate*.)

cholesterol   A type of lipid that is continually manufactured and destroyed in the body. Dietary cholesterol is consumed in food (mainly animal products). Blood levels of cholesterol, especially LDL, are often high in poorly controlled diabetes and cardiovascular disease. Cholesterol deposited in the blood vessels is a major cause of cardiovascular disease. (See also *HDLs*, *LDLs*, *VLDLs*, and *plaque*.)

cholesterol free   A food item must contain less than 2 milligrams of cholesterol and 2 grams or less of saturated fat per 50 grams of food to be labeled "cholesterol free." (See also *low cholesterol*.)

chromosomes   The coiled molecules in each cell nucleus where genetic information resides. Chromosomes contain DNA and are capable of reproducing their physical and chemical structure throughout successive cell division. (See also *DNA* and *genes*.)

chylomicrons These largest and least dense lipoproteins are formed in intestinal-wall cells following digestion and absorption of fats and are used to transport ingested fats to all body cells.

coenzyme A substance, usually made out of a vitamin, associated with many enzymes and essential for their functioning. It must be obtained from food because it cannot be manufactured by the body. (See also *enzyme*.)

cofactor An element (for example, a coenzyme) with which another must unite in order to function.

complex carbohydrate See *carbohydrate*.

coronary arteries The arteries that supply the heart muscle with oxygen and nutrients. A common site for atherosclerosis.

dehydration Loss of too much body water, causing the body to malfunction. Severe diarrhea or vomiting can cause dehydration.

DHA **(docosahexaenoic acid)** A long-chain omega-3 fatty acid found mainly in fish and marine microorganisms and plants. It and EPA (eicosapentaenoic acid) are the major reasons fish oils have beneficial effects on the cardiovascular system. As a precursor to series 3 eicosanoids, which dilate blood vessels and slow blood clotting, DHA is critical to the maintenance of normal cardiovascular health. (See also EPA.)

diabetes mellitus Diabetes is a metabolic disorder, which is characterized by elevated blood sugar levels. Diabetes occurs when the pancreas does not produce enough insulin or the cells become resistant to the effects of insulin.

DNA **(deoxyribonucleic acid)** The carrier of genetic information for all organisms (except the RNA viruses).

dyslipidemia   Inherited or acquired disorder of lipoprotein metabolism. (See also *lipoprotein*.)

EFAS **(essential fatty acids)**   The fatty acids that the body cannot synthesize but needs for normal metabolism: linoleic acid (LA) and linolenic acid (LNA). Some consider DHA (docosahexaenoic acid) and EPA (eicosapentaenoic acid) conditionally EFAS; the body can manufacture them from LA and LNA, but only at a low and potentially insufficient rate. (See also *FAS [fatty acids]*.)

electrolytes   A general term for the minerals responsible for proper fluid balance, including sodium, potassium, magnesium, calcium, and chloride.

endocrinologist   A medical doctor whose area of expertise is the endocrine system and its disorders. An endocrinologist is an important member of the medical team for anyone with diabetes.

enzyme   A protein substance that acts as a catalyst in biochemical reactions.

EPA **(eicosapentaenoic acid)**   A long-chain omega-3 fatty acid containing twenty carbon atoms ($C20:5n-3$). It and DHA (docosahexaenoic acid) are considered the major reason for fish oil's beneficial effects on the cardiovascular system. EPA is the direct precursor to series 3 eicosanoids. (See also *DHA*.)

epithelial cells   Tissue that forms the outer layer of the body's surface.

ER **(endoplasmic reticulum)**   The organelle in cells responsible for the manufacture of protein and other molecules. The ER also transports molecules made in one part of the cell to another. (See also *organelles*.)

FAS **(fatty acids)**   The basic chemical units or building blocks of lipids. They give fats their physical and biological properties. (See also EFAS [*essential fatty acids*].)

fat Also called lipid. A class of chemical compounds that contain one or more fatty acids and are insoluble in water. Fat is the principal form in which energy is stored in the body, providing nine calories per gram. Lipid classes include the fat-soluble vitamins (A, D, E, and K), sterols (including cholesterol), fatty acids, neutral fats (triglycerides), waxes, steroids, and phosphatides.

fiber Also known as roughage or bulk. Fiber is any substance made from carbohydrates that resists digestion by enzymes, reaches the colon in much the same form as it was eaten, and has some effect on gastrointestinal function. Fiber can be soluble or insoluble.

free radicals Highly reactive charged particles with an extra electron. They cause damage until they find another electron to pair with. They can initiate destructive chain reactions that cause cancer and atherosclerosis. Antioxidants provide the extra electron to stabilize free radicals.

gastrointestinal (GI) tract The long tube, extending from the mouth to the anus, through which food is taken in, digested, and excreted. Also known as the alimentary canal.

genes The encoded messages in DNA that determine a person's genetic traits. (See also *DNA* and *chromosomes*.)

GLA (gamma linolenic acid) An omega-6 fatty acid that is manufactured as a result of the first step toward the production of hormonelike substances called prostaglandins.

gluconeogenesis The process of making new glucose (from protein or the glycerol portions of triglycerides).

glucose The form of sugar found in blood; a monosaccharide (simple sugar) made up of one carbon ring.

glycemic index   An index that assigns a number from 1 to 100 to each food in ascending order as it makes blood sugar levels rise.

glycogen   A temporary storage molecule for glucose that provides energy between meals. About three-quarters of a pound of glycogen is stored in the liver and muscles, enough to keep the body fueled for half a day or so. If more carbohydrate is eaten than is needed for immediate use, the rest may be stored as glycogen.

glycolipids   Compounds of fatty acids, carbohydrate, and a nitrogen-containing base. Glycolipids are part of nerve tissues and certain cell membranes.

HDLS (high-density lipoproteins)   Particles in the bloodstream composed of triglycerides, cholesterol, and other lipids and protein (with a relatively low proportion of lipid and high proportion of protein). They carry cholesterol away from artery walls and tissues, returning it to the liver for excretion as bile. HDL levels over 35 milligrams per deciliter are generally considered beneficial to cardiovascular health.

hormones   The chemicals that transport information through the bloodstream via endocrine glands. Hormones are the main regulators of metabolism, growth and development, and reproduction.

hydrogenation   Chemically altering a substance (usually a fat) by adding hydrogen atoms to its unsaturated fatty acids. Hydrogenation turns liquid vegetable fats into more solid saturated fats and can lead to the production of trans fatty acids, which elevate blood cholesterol levels.

hyperinsulinism (also called **hyperinsulinemia**)   High levels of insulin in the blood, causing blood sugar to plummet below normal fasting levels.

hypertension   Another word for high blood pressure. Hypertension is an increase in the amount of pressure the blood exerts on the vascular walls as it travels through the cardiovascular system.

insulin   The hormone secreted by the beta cells in the islets of Langerhans in the pancreas. Insulin is responsible for regulating the metabolism of carbohydrates. High levels of insulin are associated with heart disease and syndrome X. (See also *syndrome X*.)

insulin resistance   A condition where there are not enough receptor sites on cells for glucose to enter them. Insulin is the key that unlocks the receptor sites, and if not enough insulin is secreted or the body can't use it properly, a cell can be surrounded by glucose and yet be starving. Also referred to as a decrease in insulin tolerance. (See also *syndrome X*.)

islets of Langerhans   Clusters of cells scattered throughout the pancreas that comprise its endocrine portion. There are three types of these cells: alpha, beta, and delta. Degeneration of the beta cells, which secrete insulin, is one of the causes of diabetes.

LA linoleic acid   An omega-6 fatty acid that is one of the two essential FAS (the other being linolenic acid). (See also *EFAS [essential fatty acids]*.)

LDLS (low-density lipoproteins)   Derived from VLDLS (very low-density lipoproteins), these contain large amounts of cholesterol and are associated with increased risk of heart disease. (See also *cholesterol* and *lipoprotein*.)

lipid   See *fat*.

lipoprotein   A particle of protein-coated lipid and cholesterol that is soluble in water and transports lipids in the bloodstream. Lipoproteins are classified by size, composition, and density; they include chylomicrons, HDLs, LDLs, and VLDLs. (See also *chylomicrons, HDLs, LDLs,* and *VLDLs.*)

LNA linolenic acid   An omega-3 fatty acid that is one of the two essential FAs (the other being linoleic acid). (See also *EFAs [essential fatty acids].*)

low cholesterol   A food item must contain less than 20 milligrams of cholesterol and 2 grams or less of saturated fat per 50 grams of food to be labeled "low cholesterol." (See also *cholesterol free.*)

macronutrients   The nutrients the body needs in large amounts: fat, protein, carbohydrate, and water.

metabolism   The chemical changes in living cells by which energy is provided for vital processes and activities and new material is assimilated.

micronutrients   The nutrients the body needs in relatively small amounts, including vitamins, minerals, trace minerals, and antioxidants.

mitochondria   The rounded, rod-shaped organelles where cellular respiration takes place. Here more than five hundred enzymes are involved in energy-releasing activities. (See also *organelles.*)

MUFA (monounsaturated fatty acid)   A fatty acid with only one double bond. MUFAs do not raise cholesterol levels and are associated with a decreased risk of high blood pressure. Olive oil and peanut oil are sources of monounsaturated fatty acids. (See also *PUFA [polyunsaturated fatty acid]* and *saturated fat.*)

neuropathy   Disorders affecting the nervous system, specifically the cranial or spinal nerves. Diabetic neuropathy also involves the motor and sensory nerves.

neurotransmitters   Chemicals that transmit signals between the nerve cells and the brain.

nitrogen balance   The state of equilibrium in which a person's intake of nitrogen equals his or her output (the usual state for healthy adults). Someone who has more nitrogen coming in than going out is in positive nitrogen balance; someone who has more nitrogen going out than coming in is in negative nitrogen balance. Since protein is the only macronutrient that contains nitrogen, measuring the amount of nitrogen in the blood reveals the amount of protein in the body.

nucleus   The "brain" of a cell, its largest structure. Every cell in the body (except for mature red blood cells) contains a nucleus; some have more than one. The nucleus holds the chromatids, which contain the encoded instructions for all cellular functions.

omega-3 fatty acid   An unsaturated fatty-acid molecule whose first double bond is the third carbon–carbon bond from its carbon-terminal end. Omega-3 FAs are found in fish, marine plants, and some terrestrial plants.

omega-6 fatty acid   An unsaturated fatty-acid molecule whose first double bond is the sixth carbon–carbon bond from its carbon-terminal end. Omega-6 FAs are found mainly in vegetable oils and animal fat.

organ   A group of tissues working together to perform a specific function (for example, the liver or the pancreas).

organ system   A group of organs working together and depending on each other (for example, the digestive system or the endocrine system).

organelles   Structures suspended in the cytoplasm of the cells. Organelles are like miniature organs of the body, each one performing a specialized function related to growth, repair, maintenance, and control.

oxidation   Addition of oxygen to a chemical structure. Oxidation causes rancidity in oils and may be a source of the carcinogenic properties of some oils. Oxidation makes LDL (low-density lipoproteins) particles much more likely to damage the vascular walls.

pancreas   A large organ situated behind the stomach. Its external secretion contains a variety of digestive enzymes. Its internal secretion is insulin, which is produced in the beta cells and is needed to regulate carbohydrate metabolism.

pharmacopoeia   A book, especially one published by a recognized authority like the government, that lists drugs and describes their formulas, methods of making medicinal preparations, requirements and tests for strength and purity, and related information.

phospholipids   Compounds of fatty acids, phosphoric acid, and a nitrogen-containing base. Lecithin is one of the most common phospholipids.

phytochemicals   A wide variety of naturally occurring compounds, many of which the body can use, found in plant foods. For example, polyphenols kill viruses, glutathione quenches free radicals, and pectin reduces cholesterol.

plaque   Also called an atheroma. A localized abnormal collection of fat, cholesterol, connective tissue, and calcium that occurs in the inner lining of a blood vessel wall. Large plaques can block the arteries; unstable plaques break and form blood clots.

plasma membrane   The thin structure that separates the inside of a cell from the outside.

platelets   Blood cells involved in clotting mechanisms.

PUFA **(polyunsaturated fatty acid)** A fatty acid with more than one double bond. PUFAs are liquid at room temperature and are more fragile than saturated fats and MUFAS. (See also *MUFA [monounsaturated fatty acid]* and *saturated fat*.)

rancidity An off flavor in edible oils and fats, or in manufactured food products, caused by oxidative deterioration. (See also *oxidation*.)

RDA **(recommended dietary allowance)** The levels of intake of essential nutrients judged by the Food and Nutrition Board, on the basis of scientific evidence, to be adequate to meet the minimum nutrient needs of healthy people.

receptor sites Molecules attach to these sites outside of a cell's plasma membrane which receive packages of hormones, nutrients, enzymes, neurotransmitters, and antibodies from other cells.

RNA **(ribonucleic acid)** A nucleic acid found in all living cells.

saturated fat A type of fat found in animal products, usually solid at room temperature. It tends to raise blood cholesterol levels, and a diet high in saturated fats is associated with cardiovascular disease.

simple carbohydrate See *carbohydrate*.

sterols A group of lipids that includes cholesterol and beta sitosterol, among others.

syndrome X Also called the insulin resistance syndrome. A collection of symptoms that includes high blood pressure, high triglycerides, low HDL cholesterol, decreased glucose tolerance, decreased insulin sensitivity, and abdominal obesity.

tissues Groups of cells that have the same encoded message to perform a specialized activity.

toxin A poisonous substance.

trans fatty acid An unsaturated fatty acid whose atoms are such that the molecule acts like a saturated FA. Frequently formed during hydrogenation of vegetable fats and considered dangerous to one's health.

triglyceride The most common form of fat. It is made up of three fatty acids connected to a glycerol molecule.

turbidity The degree of cloudiness or amount of stirred-up sediment in water.

type 1 diabetes Also called insulin-dependent diabetes. In this condition, the patient has high blood sugar and either cannot produce insulin or has reduced secretions of insulin from the beta cells of the pancreas. Type 1 usually occurs in younger people. (See also *diabetes mellitus*.)

type 2 diabetes Also called noninsulin-dependent diabetes. It generally occurs in adults, most often those who are overweight and have developed insulin resistance. This type makes up 90 percent of diabetes cases. (See also *diabetes mellitus*.)

veins The vessels that carry blood back to the heart. The smallest veins are called venules. (See also *arteries* and *capillaries*.)

VLDLs (very low-density lipoproteins) Lipoproteins made in the liver and responsible for transporting triglycerides and small amounts of cholesterol to tissues.

Resources

American Diabetes Association (national office)
1660 Duke St.
Alexandria, VA 22314
(800) 232-3472

Cornell University
Call Cornell University's garlic hot line for answers to your questions about garlic. Open 9 A.M. to 5 P.M. Eastern time, Monday through Friday: (800) 330-5922.

International Diabetic Athletes Association
6829 N. 12th St., Ste. 205
Phoenix, AZ 85014

FDA Center for Food Safety and Applied Nutrition
Website: http://vm.cfsn.fda.gov/label.html

U.S. Office of Disease Prevention and Health Promotion
Website: http://altmed.od.nih.gov

Sally J. Rockwell, C.N., Ph.D., Nutritionist
4703 Stone Way North
Seattle, WA 98103
(206) 547-1814
Fax: (206) 547-7696
E-mail: docrock@accessone.com
Website: www.arxc.com/doctors/rockwell.htm
If you have been diagnosed with candida or food allergies, you can call Dr. Rockwell's office for telephone counseling. You can

also request information on diabetes, hypoglycemia, whole-foods diet, and vegetarian sources of calcium. Her diet for blood sugar control is based on Dr. Elias Ilyias's 2:1 carbo:protein plan and is compatible with the basic meal plan in this book.

The Alacer Corporation

Foothills Ranch, CA 92610

(714) 454-3900

(800) 854-0249

Fax: (714) 951-7235

E-mail: @alacercorp.com

Health-food stores usually carry Alacer's E-mer'gen-C product, a vitamin supplement, or you can order it directly from Alacer. Call the toll-free number for product information. Alacer also sells Miracle Sports, a beverage that can be used to replace water and electrolytes.

Body Ecology

1266 West Paces Ferry Rd., Ste. 505

Atlanta, GA 30327

(404) 266-1366

(800) 478-3942

The company sells stevia, kefer, and essential-oil mixes to take as a supplement. Call its toll-free number for a product list.

Cheryl's Herbs

836 Hanley Ind. Ct.

St. Louis, MO 63144

(800) 231-5971

Fax: (314) 963-4454

E-mail: pawgep@aol.com

The company has a line of stevia products, including stevia leaf powder and stevia extract. Call the toll-free number for a free catalog.

Herbal Advantage, Inc.

Route 3, Box 93
Rogerville, MO 65742-9214
(800) 753-9199
Fax: (417) 753-2000
E-mail: smarsden@mail.orion.org
Website: www.HerbalAdvantage.com
Call the toll-free number for a free catalog or stevia recipe book.

Klaire Labs

Box 618
Carlsbad, CA 92008
The company carries Vitadophilus, an acidophilus product for people who are milk sensitive.

Kyolic

23501 Madero
Mission Viejo, CA 92691
Call (800) 825-7888 for a free sample of Kyolic garlic.

Multi-Pure Water Purifier

Contact: Tonya Hill at (425) 643-2240
(independent distributor)
Call for information about high-quality water purifiers for home use (for both municipal and well water).

Walnut Acres

(800) 344-9025
Call for a free catalog of organic food products, such as whole-grain breads, pasta, nut butters and seeds.

Wisdom of the Ancients—The Stevia Company
640 S. Perry Ln.
Tempe, AZ 85281
(800) 899-9908
Call for a list of the company's stevia products.

Supplement Makers
Bronson Pharmaceuticals
1945 Craig Rd.
St. Louis, MO 63146-4105
(800) 235-3200
8 A.M. to 7 P.M. Central time
Bronson's vitamins and herbals are sold only through health professionals. Call its toll-free number for the names of those who are selling the products in your area. Bronson carries such products as black currant seed oil (essential fatty acids) with vitamin E, garlic capsules, lecithin granules, chewable digestive enzymes, and buffered powdered vitamin C.

Metagenics
(800) 692-9400
(800) 338-3948
8 A.M. to 6 P.M. Pacific time
Metagenics' supplements are sold only through health professionals. Call its toll-free number for the names of those who carry the products in your area. Metagenics carries vitamins and mineral combinations, a complete line of high-quality protein powders, and enzymes. It sells chromium picolinate, buffered vitamin C, CoQ_{10}, multigenics (vitamin and mineral complex), chewable and powdered multivitamins, Omega-EFA (essential fatty acids supplement), and the intestinal flora products Ultra Bifidus and Ultra Dophilus.

Thorne Research, Inc.
4000 Highway 2 West
Dover, ID 83825
(800) 228-1966
Fax: (208) 265-2488
E-mail: info@thorne.com
Thorne vitamin, mineral, and encapsulated products are of high quality and sold only through health professionals. Call its toll-free number for the names of those who carry the products in your area. Thorne sells multivitamins, chromium picolinate (Ultrachrome), calcium magnesium citrate, and vanadium (Vonoxyl 5).

Suggested Reading Materials

Bread Machine Baking for Better Health
by Maureen B. Keane, M.S., and Daniella Chace, M.S.
Prima Publishing, 1994
This cookbook includes recipes for whole-grain breads that can be made in a bread machine or baked in an oven. There are chapters devoted to wheat-free, gluten-free, lactose-free, low-fat, and high-protein breads. The recipes for flours made from spelt, garbanzo beans, rice, soy, tapioca, and potatoes are especially useful for people with specific grain allergies.

Diabetes and Hypoglycemia
by Michael T. Murray, N.D.
Prima Publishing, 1994
Dr. Murray's book details the use of herbs, vitamins, and minerals in therapy and brings the insight only a naturopathic doctor can to natural therapies in diabetic management.

Dr. Sally's Blood Sugar Blues
by Sally Rockwell, Ph.D., and Louise Bondi
Dr. Sally has a free newsletter on blood sugar control and a list of educational materials including books, other newsletters (on food allergies and candida), games, and audio and videotapes. Call (206) 547-1814, fax (206) 547-7696, or e-mail docrock@ accessone.com. You can also visit her website at www.arxc. com/doctors/rockwell.htm.

The Encyclopedia of Natural Medicine
by Michael Murray, N.D. and Joseph Pizzorno, N.D.
Prima Publishing, 1991.

The Encyclopedia of Nutritional Supplements
by Michael Murray, N.D.
Prima Publishing, 1996

Environmental Nutrition
Call (800) 829-5384 to subscribe to this newsletter.

Fast Food Facts
by Marion J. Franz, M.S., R.D.
Chronimed Publishing, 1994

The Fast Food Guidebook
Center for Science in the Public Interest, 1991

Grains for Better Health
by Maureen B. Keane, M.S., and Daniella Chace, M.S.
Prima Publishing, 1994
This cookbook includes a wide variety of delicious recipes for
the more unusual "ancient" grains, such as amaranth, kamut,
quinoa, spelt, and teff.

Nutrition Action
This newsletter is published by the Center for Science in the
Public Interest. Written in a simple, fun to read style, it will
keep you current on new healthful food products and the latest
nutrition research. Call CSPI at (202) 332-9110 to subscribe or
write: CSPI, 1875 Connecticut Ave., NW, Ste. 300, Washington,
D.C. 20009-5728. Fax: (202) 265-4954

Optimal Wellness
by Ralph Golan, M.D.
Ballantine Books, 1995
Every household should have this book. It contains practical
alternative treatments from A to Z for more than a hundred
major health problems. Dr. Golan does a superb job of defining
the peripheral issues of blood sugar disorders, such as nutritional

deficiencies, poor digestion and assimilation, a sluggish liver, yeast overgrowth, and food allergies.

Outsmarting Diabetes
by Richard S. Beaser, M.D., with the staff of the Joslin Diabetes Center
Chronimed Publishing, 1994
This book offers guidelines for what the authors call an intensive diabetes therapy that includes insulin pumps, multiple injections, and an exercise plan. It also addresses pregnancy.

Pressure Cooking the Meatless Way—Over 125 Delicious and Nutritious Recipes for Today's Busy Cook
by Maureen B. Keane and Daniella Chace
Prima Publishing, 1996
This book offers a wide range of whole grain and legume recipes made in pressure cookers.

Smoothies for Life!
by Daniella Chace and Maureen B. Keane
Prima Publishing, 1998
Every smoothie recipe in this book has a complete nutrition analysis to help you choose those that fit into your meal plan.

The Yeast Connection
by William G. Crook, M.D.
Professional Books, 1983, 1989
Dr. Crook explains the connections among hormones, mood, yeast infections, food allergies, and blood sugar.

The What to Eat If You Have Diabetes Cookbook
by Daniella Chace and Maureen B. Keane
Contemporary Books, 1999
This book offers many delicious recipes for breakfast, lunch, dinner, and snacks. A nutritional analysis is included with every recipe. Use in conjunction with this book.

References

Abraham, A. S., Brooks, B. A., and Eylath, U. 1992. The effects of chromium supplementation on serum glucose and lipids in patients with and without non-insulin dependent diabetes. *Metabolism* 41:768–71.

Agrawal, P., Rai, V., Singh, R. B. 1996. Randomized placebo-controlled, single blind trial of holy basil leaves in patients with noninsulin-dependent diabetes mellitus. *International Journal of Clinical Pharmacological Therapy* 34(9):406–9.

American Diabetes Association. 1987. *Diabetes in the Family*. New York: Prentice Hall.

American Diabetes Association. 1987. Nutritional recommendations and principles for individuals with diabetes mellitus. *Diabetes Care* 10.

American Diabetes Association. 1987. Principles of nutrition and dietary recommendations for individuals with diabetes mellitus. *Diabetes Care* 20.

The American Society of Clinical Nutrition. 1995. The international tables of glycemic index. *American Journal of Clinical Nutrition* 62:87S–93S.

Anderson, J. W. 1977. High-polysaccharide diet studies in patients with diabetes and vascular disease. *Cereal Foods World* 22:12–22.

Anderson, J. W. 1979. High-carbohydrate, high-fiber diets for patients with diabetes. In Camerini-Davalos, R. A., and Hanover, eds. *Treatment of Early Diabetes*. New York: Plenum Medical Book Co.

Anderson, J. W., and Ward, K. 1979. High-carbohydrate, high-fiber diet for insulin-treated men with diabetes mellitus. *American Journal of Clinical Nutrition* 32:2312–21.

Anderson, R. A. 1992. Chromium, glucose tolerance and diabetes. *Biological Trace Element Research* 32:19–24.

Anderson, R. A., et al. 1987. Effects of supplemention chromium on patients with symptoms of reactive hypoglycemia. *Metabolism* 36:351–55.

Arsenio, L., et al. 1984. Hyperlipidemia, diabetes and atherosclerosis: Efficacy of treatment with pantethine. *Acta Biomed Ateneo Parmense* 55(1):25–42.

Arsenio, L., Bodria, P., Magnati, G., et al. 1986. Effectiveness of long-term treatment with pantethine in patients with dyslipidemias. *Clinical Therapeutics* 8:537–45.

Balch, J. F., and Balch, P. A. 1990. *Prescription for Nutritional Healing*. Avery Publishing Group.

Baldy, D. 1990. Effect of manganese deficiency on insulin binding, glucose transport and metabolism in rat adipocytes. *Journal of Nutrition* 120:1075–79.

Bantle, J., Swanson, J., Thomas, W., and Laine, D. 1992. Metabolic effects of dietary fructose in diabetic subjects. *Diabetes Care* 15(11):1468–76.

Beasley, J., and Swift, J. 1989. *The Kellogg Report: The Impact of Nutrition, Environment and Lifestyle on the Health of Americans*. The Institute of Health Policy and Practice, The Bard College Center. 174–90.

Behall, K. M., 1990. Effect of soluble fibers on plasma lipids, glucose tolerance, and mineral balance. *Adv. Exp. Med. Biol.* 270:7–16.

Behme, M. T. 1995. Nicotinamide and diabetes prevention. *Nutrition Reviews* 53:137–39.

Bertolini, S., et al. 1986. Lipoprotein changes induced by pantethine in hyperlipoproteinemic patients: Adults and children. *International Journal of Clinical Pharmacology, Therapy, and Toxicology* 24(11):630–37.

Bertorelli, A. M., Czarnowski-Hill, J. V. 1990. Review of present and future use of nonnutritive sweeteners. *The Diabetes Educator* 16(5):415–22.

Binaghi, P., et al. 1990. Evaluation of the cholesterol-lowering effectiveness of pantethine in women in perimenopausal age. *Minerva Medicine* 81(6):475–79.

Boyle, E., Mondschein, B., and Dash, H. 1977. Chromium depletion in the pathogenesis of diabetes and atherosclerosis. *Southern Medical Journal* 70:1449–53.

Brichard, S. M., and Henquin, J. C. 1995. The role of vanadium in the management of diabetes. *Trends in Pharmacological Sciences* 16:265–70.

Butland, B. K. 1988. Heart disease in British vegetarians. *American Journal of Clinical Nutrition* 48:830–32.

Cameron, N. E., Cotter, M. A., Dines, K. C., Robertson, S., and Cox, D. 1993. The effects of evening primrose oil on nerve function and capillarization in streptozotocin-diabetic rats: Modulation by the cyclo-oxygenase inhibitor flurbiprofen. *British Journal of Pharmacology* 109(4):972–79.

Cattin, L., et al. 1985. Treatment of hypercholesterolemia with pantethine and fenofibrate: An open randomized study on 43 subjects. *Current Therapeutic Research* 386–95.

Cavallo, M. G., Fava, D., Monetini, L., et al. 1996. Cell-mediated immune response to beta casein in recent-onset insulin-dependent diabetes: Implications for disease pathogenesis. *Lancet* 348:926–28.

Cederblad, G., Hermansson, G., and Ludvigsson, J. 1982. Plasma and urine carnitine in children with diabetes mellitus. *Clinica Chimica Acta* 125:207–17.

Chase, H. P., et al. 1991. A trial of nicotinamide in newly diagnosed insulin dependent diabetic patients: Final results. *Diabetologia* 34 (Suppl. 2):A29.

Clements, R. S., Jr. 1986. New therapies for the chronic complications of older diabetic patients. *American Journal of Medicine* 80:54–60.

Coelingh-Bennick, H. J. T., and Schreurs, W. H. P. 1975. Improvement of oral glucose tolerance in gestational diabetes. *British Medical Journal* 3:13–15.

Coggeshall, J. C., Heggers, J. P., Robson, M. C., and Baker, H. 1985. Biotin status and plasma glucose in those with diabetes. *Annals of the New York Academy of Sciences* 447:389–92.

Cohen, N., et al. 1995. Oral vanadyl sulfate improves hepatic and peripheral insulin sensitivity in patients with non-insulin-dependent diabetes mellitus. *Journal of Clinical Investigation* 95:2501–9.

Collings, A. 1989. Metabolism of cyclamate and its conversion to cyclohexylamine. *Diabetes Care* 12(1):50–55.

Consensus statement: Magnesium supplementation in the treatment of diabetes. 1996. *Diabetes Care* 19 (Suppl. 1):S93–95.

Coronel, F., et al. 1991. Treatment of hyperlipidemia in diabetic patients on dialysis with a physiological substance. *American Journal of Nephrology* 11(1):32–36.

Crapo, P. 1989. Use of alternative sweeteners in the diabetic diet. *Diabetes Care* 11(2):174–82.

Cunningham, J. J., et al. 1994. Vitamin C: An aldose reductase inhibitor that normalizes erythrocyte sorbitol in insulin-dependent diabetes mellitus. *Journal of the American College of Nutrition* 13:344–50.

Davie, S. J., Gould, B. J., and Yudkin, J. S. 1992. Effect of vitamin C on glycosylation of proteins. *Diabetes* 41:167–73.

Djurhuus, M. S., et al. 1995. Insulin increases renal magnesium excretion: A possible cause of magnesium depletion in hyperinsulinemic states. *Diabetic Medicine* 12:664–69.

Donati, C., Bertieri, R. S., and Barbi, G. 1989. Pantethine, diabetes mellitus and atherosclerosis: Clinical study of 1045 patients. *Clinical Therapeutics* 128(6):411.

Donati, C., et al. 1986. Pantethine improves the lipid abnormalities of chronic hemodialyis patients: Results of a multicenter clinical trial. *Clinical Nephrology* 25(2):70–74.

Douillet, C., Tabib, A., Bost, M., Accominotti, M., Borson-Chazot, F., and Ciavatti, M. 1996. A selenium supplement, associated or not with vitamin E, delays early renal lesions in experimental diabetes in rats. *Proceedings of the Society for Experimental Biology and Medicine* 211(4):323–31.

El-Enien, A. M. A., et al. 1983. The role of nicotinic acid and inositol hexaniacinate as anticholesterolemic and antilipidemic agents. *Nutrition Reports International* 28:899–911.

Elliot, R. B., and Chase, H. P. 1991. Prevention or delay of type 1 (insulin-dependent) diabetes mellitus in children using nicotinamide. *Diabetologia* 34:362–65.

Elliot, R. B., and Pilcher, C. C. 1991. Prevention of diabetes in normal school children. *Diabetes Research and Clinical Practice* 14:S85.

Elliot, R. B., Pilcher, C. C., Fergusson, D. M., and Steward, A. W. 1996. A population-based strategy to prevent insulin-dependent diabetes using nicotinamide. *Journal of Pediatric Endocrinology and Metabolism* 9:501–9.

Ellis, J. M., Folkers, K., Minadeo, M., et al. 1991. A deficiency of vitamin B_6 is a plausible molecular basis of the retinopathy of patients with diabetes mellitus. *Biochemical and Biophysical Research Communications* 179:615–19.

Erickson, J., and Kohvakka, A. 1995. Magnesium and ascorbic acid supplementation in diabetes mellitus. *Annals of Nutrition and Metabolism* 39:217–23.

Estrada, D. E., Ewart, H. S., Tsakiridis, T., Volchuk, A., Ramlal, T., Tritschler, H., and Klip. 1996. Stimulation of glucose uptake by the natural coenzyme alpha-lipoic acid/thioctic acid: Participation of elements of the insulin signaling pathway. *Diabetes* 45(12):1798–1804.

Foster, H. 1987. Diabetes mellitus and low environmental magnesium levels. *Lancet* 12(2):559–633.

Franz, M. J., Horton, E. S., Bantle, J. P., Beebe, C. A., and Brunzell, J. 1994. Nutrition principles for the management of diabetes and related complications. *Diabetes Care* 17(5):490–518.

Fraser, G. E. 1988. Determinants of ischemic heart disease in Seventh-Day Adventists. *American Journal of Clinical Nutrition* 48:833–36.

Freund, H. 1979. Chromium deficiency during total parenteral nutrition. *Journal of the American Medical Association* 241(5):496–98.

Fuller, C. J., Chandalia, M., Garg, A., Grundy, S. M., and Jialal, I. 1996. Alpha tocopheryl acetate supplementation at pharmacologic doses decreases low-density-lipoprotein oxidative susceptibility but not protein glycation in patients with diabetes mellitus. *American Journal of Clinical Nutrition* 65(5):753–59.

Gaddi, A., Descovich, G., Noseda, et al. 1984. Controlled evaluation of pantethine, a natural hypolipidemic compound, in patients with different forms of hyperlipoproteinemia. *Atherosclerosis* 50:73–83.

Gale, E. A. 1996. Molecular mechanisms of beta-cell destruction in IDDM: the role of nicotinamide. *Hormone Research* 45:39–43.

Gale, E. A. 1996. Theory and practice of nicotinamide trials in pretype 1 diabetes. *Journal of Pediatric Endocrinology and Metabolism* 9:375–79.

Geil, P. B., and Anderson, J. W. 1994. Nutrition and health implications of dry beans: A review. *Journal of the American College of Nutrition* 13(6):548–49.

Gensini, G. F., et al. 1985. Changes in fatty acid composition of the single platelet phospholipids induced by pantethine treatment. *International Clinical and Pharmacological Research Journal* 5(5):309–18.

Gerstein, H. C. 1994. Cow's milk exposure and type 1 diabetes mellitus: A critical review of the current literature. *Diabetes Care* 17:13–19.

Gerstein, H. C., et al. 1996. Rationale and design of a large study to evaluate the renal and cardiovascular effects of an ACE inhibitor and vitamin E in high-risk patients with diabetes. The Micro-Hope study. Microalbuminuria, cardiovascular, and renal outcomes. Heart outcomes prevention evaluation. *Diabetes Care* 19(11):1225–28.

Goday, A., et al. 1993. Effects of a short prednisone regime at clinical onset of IDDM. *Diabetes Research and Clinical Practice* 20:39–46.

Greco, A. V., et al. 1992. Effect of propionyl-L-carnitine in the treatment of diabetic angiopathy: Controlled double blind trial versus placebo. *Drugs in Experimental and Clinical Research* 18(2):69–80.

Greenbaum, C. J., Kahn, S. E., and Palmer, J. P. 1996. Nicotinamide's effect on glucose metabolism in subjects at risk for IDDM. *Diabetes* 45:501–9.

Gregersen, G., et al. 1983. Oral supplementation of myoinositol: Effects on peripheral nerve function in human diabetics and on the concentration in plasma, erythrocytes, urine and muscle tissue in human diabetics and normals. *Acta Neurologica Scandinavica* 67(3):164–72.

Haglund, B., et al. 1996. Evidence of a relationship between childhood-onset type 1 diabetes and low groundwater concentration of zinc. *Diabetes Care* 19(8):873–75.

Haire-Joshu, D. 1992. *Management of Diabetes Mellitus: Perspectives of Care Across the Life Span.* St. Louis, MO: Mosby Year Book.

Harland, B. F., and Harden-Williams, B. A. 1994. Is vanadium of human nutritional importance yet? *Journal of the American Dietetic Association* 94(8):891–94.

Haylock, S. 1983. Separation of biologically active chromium-containing complexes from yeast extract and other sources of glucose tolerance factor (GTF) activity. *Journal of Inorganic Biochemistry* 18(3):195–211.

Head, Kathleen. 1997. Type 1 diabetes: Prevention of the disease and its complications. *Alternative Medicine Review* 2(4):256–81.

Herskowitz, R. D., et al. 1989. Pilot trial to prevent type 1 diabetes: Progression to overt IDDM despite oral nicotinamide. *Journal of Autoimmunity* 2:733–37.

Hiramatsu, K., Nozaki, H., and Arimori, S. 1981. Influence of pantethine on platelet volume, microviscosity, lipid composition and functions in diabetes mellitus with hyperlipidemia. *Tokai Journal of Experimental and Clinical Medicine* 6(1):49–57.

Hollenbeck, C. B., Leklem, J. E., Riddle, M. C., and Connor, W. E. 1983. The composition and nutritional adequacy of subject-selected high-carbohydrate, low-fat meal plans in insulin-dependent diabetes mellitus. *American Journal of Clinical Nutrition* 38:41–51.

Horwitz, D., McLane, M., and Kobe, P. 1988. Response to single dose of aspartame or saccharin by NIDDM patients. *Diabetes Care* 11(3):230–34.

Jain, S. K., McVie, R., Jaramillo, J. J., Palmer, M., and Smith, T. 1996. Effect of modest vitamin E supplementation on blood glycated hemoglobin and triglyceride levels and red cell indices in type 1 diabetic patients. *Journal of the American College of Nutrition* 15(5):458–61.

Jenkins, D. J., et al. 1980. Diabetic diets: High carbohydrate combined with high fiber. *American Journal of Clinical Nutrition* 33(8):1729–33.

Jenkins, D. J., et al. 1994. Low glycemic index: Lente carbohydrates and physiological effects of altered food frequency. *American Journal of Clinical Nutrition* 59(3):706S–709S.

Jones, C. L., and Gonzales, V. 1978. Pyridoxine deficiency: A new factor in diabetic neuropathy. *Journal of the American Podiatry Association* 68:646–53.

Karjalainen, J., Martin, J., Knip, M., et al. 1992. A bovine albumin peptide as a possible trigger of insulin-dependent diabetes. *New England Journal of Medicine* 327(5):302–7.

Kay, R., Grobin, W., and Trace, N. 1981. Diets rich in natural fiber improve carbohydrate tolerance in maturity onset, non-insulin dependent diabetes. *Diabetologia* 20:12–23.

Kestin, M., Rouse, I., Correl, R., and Nestel, P. 1989. Cardiovascular disease risk factors in free-living men: Comparison of two prudent diets, one based on lactoovovegetarianism and the other allowing lean meat. *American Journal of Clinical Nutrition* 50:280–87.

Kiehm, T. G., Anderson, J. W., and Ward, K. 1976. Beneficial effects of a high-carbohydrate, high-fiber diet on a hyperglycemic diabetic man. *American Journal of Clinical Nutrition* 28(8):895–99.

Kirkeeide, R., Brand, R., and Gould, K. L. 1990. Can lifestyle changes reverse coronary heart disease? *Lancet* 336(8708):129–33.

Kishi, T., et al. 1976. Bioenergetics in clinical medicine, XI studies on coenzyme Q and diabetes mellitus. *Journal of Medicine* 7:307.

Kodentsova, V. M., Vrzhesinskaia, O. A., Sokol'nikov, A. A., et al. 1994. Vitamin metabolism in children with insulin-dependent diabetes mellitus. Effect of length of illness, severity and degree of disruption of substance metabolism. *Voprosky Meditsinskoi Khimii* 40:33–38.

Kodentsova, V. M., Vrzhesinskaia, O. A., Sokol'nikov, A. A., et al. 1993. Metabolism of riboflavin and B group vitamins functionally bound to it in insulin-dependent diabetes mellitus. *Voprosky Meditsinskoi Khimii* 39:33–36.

Koutsikos, D., Agroyannis, B., and Tzanatos-Exarchou, H. 1990. Biotin for diabetic peripheral neuropathy. *Biomedicine and Pharmacotherapy* 44:511–14.

Kowluru, R. A., Kern, T. S., and Engerman, R. L. 1997. Abnormalities of retinal metabolism in diabetes or experimental galactosemia. IV Antioxidant defense system. *Free Radical Biology and Medicine* 22(4):587–92.

Kuznetsov, N. S., Abulela, A. M., and Neskromnyi, V. N. 1994. The comparative evaluation of the efficacy of tocopherol acetate in the combined treatment of patients with hypertension and diabetes mellitus. *Lik Sprava* (9–12):133–36.

Lazarow, A., Liambies, L., and Tausch, A. J. 1950. Protection against diabetes with nicotinamide. *Journal of Laboratory and Clinical Medicine* 36:249–58.

Leeds, A. 1981. Legume diets for those with diabetes? *Journal of Plant Foods* 3:219–23.

Lefavi, R. G., Anderson, R. A., Keith, R. E., Wilson, G. D., McMillan, J. L., and Stone, M. H. 1992. Efficacy of chromium supplementation in athletes: Emphasis on anabolism. *International Journal of Sport Nutrition* 2:111–22.

Lefebvre, P. J., Paolisso, G., and Scheen, A. J. 1994. Magnesium and glucose metabolism. *Therapie* 49(1):1–7.

Leslie, D. G., and Elliot, R. B. 1994. Early environmental events as a cause of IDDM. *Diabetes* 43: 843–50.

Levy-Marchal, C., Karjalainen, J., Dubois, F., et al. 1995. Antibodies against bovine albumin and other diabetic markers in French children. *Diabetes Care* 18:1089–94.

Lewis, C. M., et al. 1992. Double-blind randomized trial of nicotinamide on early onset diabetes. *Diabetes Care* 15:121–23.

Mandrup, Paulsen, T., et al. 1993. Nicotinamide in the prevention of insulin dependent diabetes mellitus. *Diabetes Metabolism Review* 9:295–309.

Manganese and glucose tolerance. 1968. *Nutrition Reviews* 26:207–10.

Mann, J. 1985. Fiber and diabetes. *Diabetes Care* 8:192–93.

Manna, R., et al. 1992. Nicotinamide treatment in subjects at high risk of developing IDDM improves insulin secretion. *British Journal of Clinical Practice* 46:177–179.

Mathieu, C., Waer, M., Casteels, K., et al. 1995. Prevention of type 1 diabetes in NOD mice by nonhypercalcemic doses of a new structural analog of 1,25-dihydroxy-vitamin D3, KH1060. *Endocrinology* 136(3):866–72.

Mendola, G., Casamitjana, R., and Gomis, R. 1989. Effect of nicotinamide therapy upon beta-cell function in newly diagnosed type 1 (insulin-dependent) diabetic patients. *Diabetologia* 32:A160.

Mertz, W. 1993. Chromium in human nutrition: A review. *Journal of Nutrition* 123:626–33.

Mertz, W., and Schwartz, K. 1959. Chromium (III) and the glucose tolerance factor. *Archives of Biochemistry and Biophysics* 85:292–95.

Mijac, V., Arrieta, J., Mendt, C., et al. 1995. Role of environmental factors in the development of insulin-dependent diabetes mellitus (IDDM) in insulin-dependent Venezuelan children. *Investigative Clinica* 36:73–82.

Miller, S., and Frattali, V. 1989. Saccharin. *Diabetes Care* 12(1):74–80.

Mistura, L., et al. 1987. Prednisone treatment in newly diagnosed type 1 diabetic children: One-year follow-up. *Diabetes Care* 10:39–43.

Mooradian, A. D., and Morley, J. 1987. Micronutrient status in diabetes mellitus. *American Journal of Clinical Nutrition* 45(5):877–95.

Mooradian, A. D., et al. 1994. Selected vitamins and minerals in diabetes. *Diabetes Care* 17:464–79.

Mossop, R. T. 1983. Effects of chromium (III) on fasting blood glucose, cholesterol and cholesterol HDL levels in those with diabetes. *Central African Journal of Medicine* 29:80–82.

Murray and Pizzorno. 1991. Patients with glucose tolerance impairment. *Takashima Journal of Experimental Medicine* 37.

Nagamatsu, M., Nickander, K. K., Schmelzer, J. D., Raya, A., Wittrock, D. A., Tritschler, H., and Low, P. A. 1995. Lipoic acid improves nerve blood flow, reduces oxidative stress and improves distal nerve conduction in experimental diabetic neuropathy. *Diabetes Care* 18(8):1160–67.

Nickander, K. K., McPhee, B. R., Low, P. A., and Tritschler, H. 1996. Alpha-lipoic acid: Antioxidant potency against lipid peroxidation of neutral tissues in vitro and implications for diabetic neuropathy. *Free Radical Biology and Medicine* 21(5):631–39.

O'Hara, J., Jolly, P. N., and Nicol, C. G. 1988. The therapeutic effect of inositol nicotinate (Hexopal) in intermittent claudication: A controlled trial. *British Journal of Clinical Practice* 42:377–83.

Packer, L., Witt, E. H., and Tritschler, H. J. 1995. Alpha-lipoic acid as a biological antioxidant. *Free Radical Biology and Medicine* 19(2):227–50.

Paolisso, G. 1995. Metabolic benefits deriving from chronic vitamin C supplementation in aged non-insulin dependent diabetics. *Journal of the American College of Nutrition* 14(4):387–92.

Paolisso, G., et al. 1984. Pharmacological doses of vitamin E improve insulin action in healthy subjects and non-insulin-dependent diabetic patients. *American Journal of Clinical Nutrition* 3:351–56.

Paolisso, G., and Barbagallo, M. 1997. Hypertension, diabetes mellitus and insulin resistance: The role of intracellular magnesium. *American Journal of Hypertension* 10(3):368–70.

Paolisso, G., D'Amore, A., Giugliano, D., Ceriello, A., Varricchio, M., and D'Onofrio, F. 1993. Pharmacologic doses of vitamin E improve insulin action in healthy subjects and non-insulin dependent diabetic patients. *American Journal of Clinical Nutrition* 57(5):650–56.

Paolisso, G., and Ravussin, E. 1995. Intracellular magnesium and insulin resistance: Results in Pima Indians and Caucasians. *Journal of Clinical Endocrinology and Metabolism* 80(4):1382–85.

Paolisso, G., Scheen, A., D'onofrio, F., and Lefebvre, P. 1990. Magnesium and glucose homeostasis. *Diabetologia* 339:511—14.

Paolisso, G., Sgambato, Gambardella, A., et al. 1992. Daily magnesium supplements improve glucose handling in elderly subjects. *American Journal of Clinical Nutrition* 55:1161—67.

Phillips, R., and Snowdon, D. 1983. Association of meat and coffee use with cancers of the bowel, breast and prostate among Seventh-Day Adventists: Preliminary results. *Cancer Research* 45 (Suppl):2403—08.

Porikos, K., and Koopmans, H. 1988. The effect of non-nutritive sweeteners on body weight in rats. *Appetite* 11.

Pozzilli, P., et al. 1994. Combination of nicotinamide and steroid versus nicotinamide in recent onset IDDM. *Diabetes Care* 17:897—900.

Pozzilli, P., and Andreani, D. 1993. The potential role of nicotinamide in the secondary prevention of IDDM. *Diabetes/Metabolism Reviews* 9:219—30.

Pozzilli, P., Browne, P. D., and Kolb, H. 1996. Meta-analysis of nicotinamide treatment in patients with recent-onset IDDM. The nicotinamide trialists. *Diabetes Care* 19(12):1357—63.

Pozzilli, P., Visalli, N., Boccuni, M. L., et al. 1995. Adjuvant therapies in recent-onset type 1 diabetes at diagnosis and insulin requirements after 2 years. *Diabetes/Metabolism Reviews* 21:47—49.

Prisco, D., et al. 1987. Effect of oral treatment with pantethine on platelet and plasma phospholipids in a hyperlipoproteinemia. *Angiology* 38(3):241—47.

Rabinowitz, M. B., et al. 1983. Effect of chromium and yeast supplementation on carbohydrate metabolism in diabetic men. *Diabetes Care* 6:319–27.

Reddi, A., De Angelis, B., Frank, O., et al. 1988. Biotin supplementation improves glucose and insulin tolerances in genetically diabetic mice. *Life Sciences* 42(13):1323–30.

Reddy, S., Bibby, N. J., Wu, D., et al. 1995. A combined casein-free-nicotinamide meal plan prevents diabetes in the NOD mouse with minimum insulitis. *Diabetes Research and Clinical Practice* 29:83–92.

Rieder, H. P., Berger, W., and Friedrich, R. 1980. Vitamin status in diabetic neuropathy (thiamine, riboflavin, pyridoxine, cobalamin and tocopherol). *Zeitschrift fur Ernahrungswissenschaft* 19:1–13.

Rubin, R. J., et al. 1994. Health care expenditures for people with diabetes mellitus. *Journal of Clinical Endocrinology and Metabolism* 78:809A–F.

Rubinstein, A. H., Levin, N. W., and Elliot, G. A. 1962. Manganese-induced hypoglycemia. *Lancet* 2:1348–51.

Salmerón, J., and Willett, W. C. 1997. Fiber intake and risk of developing non-insulin dependent diabetes mellitus. *Journal of American Medical Association* 277:472–77.

Saukkonen, T., Savilahti, E., Landin-Olsson, M., and Dahlquist, G. 1995. IgA bovine serum albumin antibodies are increased in newly diagnosed patients with insulin-dependent diabetes mellitus, but the increase is not an independent factor for diabetes. *Acta Paediatrica* 84:1258–61.

Saukkonen, T., Savilahti, E., Madascy, L., et al. 1996. Increased frequency of IgM antibodies to cow's milk proteins in Hungarian children with newly diagnosed insulin-dependent diabetes mellitus. *European Journal of Pediatrics* 155:885–89.

Schatz, D. A., Rogers, D. G., and Brouhard, B. H. 1996. Prevention of insulin-dependent diabetes mellitus: An overview of three trials. *Cleveland Clinic Journal of Medicine* 63:270–74.

Schleicher, E. D., Wagner, E., and Nerlich, A. G. 1997. Increased accumulation of the glycoxidation product N (epsilon)-(carboxymethyl) lysine in human tissues in diabetes and aging. *Journal of Clinical Investigation* 99(3):468–75.

Schmerthaner, G. 1995. Progress in the immunointervention of type-I diabetes mellitus. *Hormone and Metabolic Research* 27:547–54.

Secchi, A., et al. 1990. Prednisone administration in recent-onset type 1 diabetes. *Journal of Autoimmunity* 3:593–600.

Seghieri, G., et al. 1994. Renal excretion of ascorbic acid in insulin dependent diabetes mellitus. *International Journal for Vitamin and Nutrition Research* 64:119–24.

Shigeta, Y., Izumi, K., and Abe, H. 1966. Effect of coenzyme Q_7 treatment on blood sugar and ketone bodies of those with diabetes. *Journal of Vitaminology* 12:293.

Silverstein, J., et al. 1988. Immunosuppression with azathioprine and prednisone in recent-onset insulin-dependent diabetes mellitus. *New England Journal of Medicine* 319:599–604.

Simpson, H. C. R., Simpson, R. W., and Lousley, S. 1981. A high-carbohydrate leguminous-fiber diet improves all aspects of diabetic control. *Lancet* 1(8210):1-5.

Sinclair, A. J., et al. 1994. Low plasma ascorbate levels in patients with type 2 diabetes mellitus consuming adequate dietary vitamin C. *Diabetic Medicine* 11(9):893–98.

Sinclair, A. J., et al. 1992. Modulators of free radical activity in diabetes mellitus: Role of ascorbic acid. *Exs* 62:342–52.

Solomon, L. R., and Cohen, K. 1989. Erythrocyte 2 transport and metabolism and effects of vitamin B$_6$ therapy in type 2 diabetes mellitus. *Diabetes* 38:881–86.

Spriestma, J. E., and Schuitemaker, G. E. 1994. Reducing insulin production can prevent diabetes. *Medical Hypotheses* 42(1):15–23.

Stone, D., and Connow, W. E. 1963. The prolonged effects of a low-cholesterol, high-carbohydrate diet on the serum lipids in diabetic patients. *Diabetes* 12:127.

Striffler, J. S., Law, J. S., Polansky, M. M., Bhathena, S. J., and Anderson, R. A. 1995. Chromium improves insulin response to glucose in rats. *Metabolism* 44(10):1314–20.

Sweetner Blending: How sweet it is! How combinations of sweeteners recreate the taste of sucrose in reduced-sugar food products. 1994. *Journal of the American Dietetic Association* 94(5):498.

Taboga, C., Tonutti, L., and Noacco, C. 1994. Residual b cell activity and insulin requirements in insulin-dependent diabetic patients treated from the beginning with high doses of nicotinamide. A two-year follow-up. *Recenti Progressi in Medicina* 85:513–16.

Truswell, A. S. 1994. Food carbohydrates and plasma lipids: An update. *American Journal of Clinical Nutrition* 59 (3 Suppl):710S–18S.

Vaarala, O., Klemetti, P., Savilahti, E., et al. 1996. Cellular immune response to cow's milk beta-lactoglobulin in patient with newly diagnosed IDDM. *Diabetes* 45:178–82.

Vague, P., Picq, R., Bernal, M., et al. 1989. Effect of nicotinamide treatment on the residual insulin secretion in type 1 (insulin-dependent) patients. *Diabetologia* 32:316–21.

Vahasalo, P., et al. 1996. Relation between antibodies to islet cell antigens, other autoantigens, and cow's milk proteins in diabetic children and unaffected siblings at the clinical manifestation of IDDM. The childhood diabetes in Finland study group. *Autoimmunity* 23(3):165–74.

Vahouny, G., and Kritchevsky, D. 1982. *Dietary Fiber in Health and Disease*. New York: Plenum Press.

Vialettes, B., et al. 1990. A preliminary multicentre study of the treatment of recently diagnosed type 1 diabetes by combination nicotinamide-cyclosporin therapy. *Diabetic Medicine* 7:731–35.

Wang, H., et al. 1995. Experimental and clinical studies on the reduction of erythrocyte sorbitol-glucose ratios by ascorbic acid in diabetes mellitus. *Diabetes Research and Clinical Practice* 28:1–8.

Warshaw, H. S., and Powers, M. A. 1993. Ingredients that replace fat: Their role in today's foods and challenges in educating people with diabetes. *Diabetes Educator* 19(5):419–30.

Welihinda, J., Arvidson, G., Gylfe, E., et al. 1982. The insulin-releasing activity of the tropical plant Momordica charantia. *Acta Biologica et Medica Germanica* 41:1229–40.

Welihinda, J., Karunanaya, E. H., Sheriff, M. H. R., et al. 1986. Effect of Momordica charantia on the glucose tolerance in maturity onset diabetes. *Journal of Ethnopharmacology* 17:277–82.

Welsh, A. L., and Ede, M. 1961. Inositol hexanicotinate for improved nicotinic acid therapy. *International Records of Medicine* 174:9–15.

White, J. R., and Campbell, R. K. 1993. Magnesium and diabetes: A review. *Annals of Pharmacotherapy* 27:775–80.

Wimhurst, J. M., and Manchester, K. L. 1972. Comparison of ability of magnesium and manganese to activate the key enzymes of glycolysis. *FEBS Letters* 27:321–26.

Zhang, H., et al. 1996. A high biotin diet improves the impaired glucose tolerance of long-term spontaneously hyperglycemic rats with noninsulin-dependent diabetes mellitus. *Journal of Nutr. Sci-Vitaminol* 42(6):517–26.

Index

Veins, 21
Viruses, 163, 169–71
Vitamins
B vitamins, 102–13
in beans, 54
vitamin A, 98–99
vitamin C, 113–15
vitamin D, 99–100
vitamin E, 100–1
vitamin K, 101
Volatile organic compounds, 198

Walnut oil, 82
Warning signs of diabetes, 165
Water, 197–208
bottled, 201–2
contaminants in, 198–201
health benefits of, 197–98
purification systems, 204–7
sources, 207–8

standards for drinking water,
202–4
from wells, 207–8
Water softeners, 207
Water-soluble vitamins, 102–17
Weight loss
habits for, 151–52
as warning sign for diabetes, 165
*The What to Eat if You Have Diabetes
Cookbook*, 131
White rice, 50
Whole foods, defined, 49–50
Whole milk, 82. *See also* Milk
Whole wheat, 49

Xylitol, 232–33

Yogurt, 48, 93, 252

Zinc, 123–24